'This book is an essential buy for undergraduate and postgraduate physiotherapists, osteopaths and chiropractors looking to develop their manual therapy skills. I have attended the authors' Chiropractic and Osteopathic Manipulation course, and the book complements it perfectly with clear illustrations and descriptions of the techniques they taught, along with enhanced theoretical knowledge to enable their safe and effective application. I will certainly be using this book to facilitate my continued clinical practice.'

*– Joe Lewis, BSc, MCSP, HCPC, Premier League Football Physiotherapist*

'A remarkable addition to anyone's library who wishes to further their understanding and performance of the techniques they are utilizing.'

*– Cody Phillips, PTA Director of Social Networking*
*at American Musculoskeletal Institute*

'A much-needed compendium...which delivers a greater body of knowledge and practical skills to any practitioner of manual manipulation.'

*– Ulrik Sandstrom, BSc, DC, ICCSD, FRCC, FBCA, FEAC, Elite Sports*
*Chiropractor and Fellow of the Royal College of Chiropractors*

# Osteopathic and Chiropractic Techniques for Manual Therapists

A Comprehensive Guide to Spinal
and Peripheral Manipulations

*Jimmy Michael, Giles Gyer and Ricky Davis*
*Foreword by Ulrik Sandstrom*

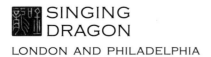 SINGING
DRAGON
LONDON AND PHILADELPHIA

First published in 2017
by Singing Dragon
an imprint of Jessica Kingsley Publishers
73 Collier Street
London N1 9BE, UK
and
400 Market Street, Suite 400
Philadelphia, PA 19106, USA

*www.singingdragon.com*

**Library of Congress Cataloging in Publication Data**
Names: Michael, Jimmy, author. | Gyer, Giles, author. | Davis, Ricky, author.
Title:
Osteopathic and Chiropractic Techniques for Manual Therapists: A Comprehensive
Guide to Spinal and Peripheral Manipulations / Jimmy
    Michael, Giles Gyer, and Ricky Davis.
Description: London ; Philadelphia : Jessica Kingsley Publishers, 2017. |
    Includes bibliographical references and index.
Identifiers: LCCN 2016047241 (print) | LCCN 2016048874 (ebook) | ISBN
    9781848193260 (alk. paper) | ISBN 9780857012814 (ebook)
Subjects: | MESH: Manipulation, Osteopathic--methods | Manipulation,
    Chiropractic--methods | Musculoskeletal Diseases--therapy
Classification: LCC RZ342 (print) | LCC RZ342 (ebook) | NLM WB 940 | DDC
    615.5/33--dc23
LC record available at https://lccn.loc.gov/2016047241

**British Library Cataloguing in Publication Data**
A CIP catalogue record for this book is available from the British Library

ISBN 978 1 84819 326 0
eISBN 978 0 85701 281 4

Printed and bound in China

# Contents

# Foreword

Manipulation in its many forms has been associated with chiropractic and osteopathy since their inception. Throughout the last century, a huge number of techniques have been developed and increasingly shared between the two professions, and this book is a much-needed compendium for the modern manual practitioner. Technique choices are driven by a need to change function, and having a toolbox full of manipulative techniques drives a tailor-made approach to each patient rather than a 'one size fits all'. We should all continue to learn, and those of us with significant experience often learn more from our allied professions than our own.

I am delighted to see the thoroughness of application of both spinal and extremity techniques in this book; these will help students of the craft as well as provide new techniques and inspiration for experienced clinicians. The book does not solely present techniques, but also offers a thorough and well-referenced review of the literature on the neurophysiology of manipulation, patient safety and contraindications, as well as anatomical and functional considerations on, for example, fascia and disc pathology. The reference lists at the end of each chapter are an invaluable source of further information, and show the vast scope of material the authors have reviewed for this book.

Having worked in elite sports for 25 years, including two Olympic Games, and seen some of the world's best chiropractors, osteopaths and physiotherapists in action, it is becoming increasingly clear to me that we should learn and teach each other's best techniques. We all adapt techniques to suit our own physiology and that of the patient in front of us, and it is often easy to fall into the trap of sticking to your five best manipulations. This book has brought some new and very useful additions to my skillset and will, I'm certain, continue to inspire further expansion of my repertoire. This can only benefit my existing and future patients. I congratulate the authors on their foresight and collaborative effort in producing this book, which delivers a greater body of knowledge and practical skills to any practitioner of manual manipulation.

*Ulrik Sandstrom, BSc, DC, ICCSD, FRCC, FBCA, FEAC*
*Elite Sports Chiropractor, International Lecturer, and Fellow of the*
*British Chiropractic Association, the Royal College of Chiropractors*
*and the European Academy of Chiropractic*

# Acknowledgements

With special thanks to the following clinicians from across the world, whose help and contributions to this text have been invaluable.

**Chapter contribution:**

Dr James Inklebarger, MD, MLCOM, MFSEM, Dip.SM, GB & I DM-Smed – United States of America

**Technique contributions:**

Mr Dave Farrelly, BSc (Hons) Osteopathy – Singapore

Dr Alison Lewis, BSc (Hons) Osteopathy – Australia

Mr Andrew Johnson, MOst Osteopathy – UK

Dr Steffi Warnock, DC MChiro, Master of Chiropractic – Ireland

Dr Robert Beaven, DC MChiro, Master of Chiropractic – UK

Dr David Elliott, DC MChiro, Master of Chiropractic – UK

Dr Iain Crombie, DC MChiro, Master of Chiropractic – UK

Mr Eyal Cohen, Sports Therapist – Israel

Special thanks to:

Mr Ethan Gyer – UK

Miss Emilia Michael – UK

Miss Esmée Gyer – UK

Miss Gabriella Michael – UK

# Disclaimer

To the fullest extent of the law, neither the publisher nor the authors assume any liability for any injury and/or damage to persons or property incurred as a result of the instructions or ideas contained in the material herein.

This field is constantly evolving as new research and experience broadens our knowledge. As a result, changes in professional practice may be necessary. Practitioners and researchers should rely on their own expertise in evaluating and using any information included in this book. They should be mindful of their own safety as well as the safety of others in their care.

With respect to any techniques identified, readers are advised to research the most current information available on procedures, dosage, method and duration of treatment, and contraindications. It is the responsibility of practitioners to provide the appropriate treatment for their patients, taking into account all the necessary safety precautions.

Over decades, therapies have blended, and, regardless of therapeutic title, we are all using, to an extent, similar techniques just with differing philosophies. Spinal manipulation is utilised worldwide as an effective way to treat musculoskeletal pain and dysfunction; this book aims merely to present effective techniques from our professions and should not be used unless you have the relevant training and qualifications within manipulative therapy.

# Introduction

The use of spinal manipulation techniques within manual therapy is as old as manual therapy itself. In writing this book, we looked at combining knowledge and skill with the aim to help promote best practice, safe and effective technique, and overall improvement in patient care, regardless of professional title and philosophical background. This is a technique book written by osteopaths and chiropractors for manual therapists who have the skill and training in using spinal manipulation. This book does not replace the high level of training that these professions undertake, but gives you an insight into the most effective techniques used within clinical practice, and, in the following sections, an insight into the background and history of the two professions.

Osteopathy and chiropractic are two of the most popular forms of manual therapy. Both medical systems share a common origin, having emerged during the late 19th century with a remarkably similar disease theory. They bear many striking similarities and meet at several common points (Pettman, 2007). In many cases, they even use similar techniques to treat similar conditions. However, due to the decisions made by the earlier pioneers, osteopathy and chiropractic have evolved into two separate disciplines and can be quite different in their modern forms. Today they have a particular degree of multiplicity and complexity (Klein, 1998).

In this chapter, we discuss the basic principles of osteopathy and chiropractic, their origins (i.e. how they came to exist but diverged into two separate systems), their similarities and differences, and their therapeutic scope.

## Osteopathy

Osteopathy, also known as osteopathic medicine, is a form of manual therapy that addresses the abnormalities of structure and function to aid the body's self-healing, self-regulating mechanisms. The therapy generates its beneficial effects by stretching, massaging, and moving a patient's bones, muscles and joints. In brief, it is a patient-centric, hands-on approach to health care with a strong manual component (Paulus, 2013).

Osteopathy utilises the power of human touch in the diagnosis and treatment of a wide range of musculoskeletal conditions, including back and neck pain, shoulder pain, arthritis, osteoarthritis, postural strain, sciatica and sporting injuries. The therapy is also used in the treatment of a number of functional problems that do not directly involve bones and joints, such as headaches, migraines, otitis media, breathing disorders, menstrual problems and digestive disorders (Line and Embase, 2010).

### Origin

Dr Andrew Taylor Still, a former US Army physician, first developed the principles and philosophies of osteopathy in the mid-1800s. In his early life, he was a dedicated practitioner of orthodox medicine. However, he lost his faith in the conventional medical practices of his time after a series of tragic events overtook his loved ones (Pettman, 2007). Incensed by his inability to save his wife and children with what he had been taught, he began to seriously question the effectiveness of mainstream treatments such as purging, blistering, bloodletting and rectal feeding (Baer, 1987; Tan and Zia, 2007).

After relentless research and study, Dr Still concluded that most of the diseases occur due to damaged articulations or faulty 'lesions' in the muscular and skeletal systems, specifically in the spine and its associated musculature. As a result, he began to slowly conceive a thought that traditional bone setting could cure diseases by restoring normal function of structures in the musculoskeletal system (Still, 1908; Ward, 2015). This theory ultimately led him to raise the banner of a new medical system known as Osteopathy in 1874 (Pettman, 2007).

Dr Still met with much resistance, however, due to his unpopular belief that bone setting could cure disease, and he was even denied the opportunity to present his philosophies at Baker University in Baldwin, Kansas. He then moved to Kirksville, Missouri, and founded the first independent school of osteopathy in 1892, naming it the American School of Osteopathy (Tan and Zia, 2007).

Soon after the opening of the first school, many osteopaths, both accredited and non-accredited American Osteopathic Association (AOA) graduates, came to live and practise osteopathy in the major UK cities. They helped establish the British Osteopathic Association in 1903 as a British branch of AOA. The first school of osteopathy in the UK, the British School of Osteopathy (BSO), was founded in 1917 by John Martin Littlejohn, a student of Dr Still, who had been a lecturer at the American School of Osteopathy (Miller, 1998; Pettman, 2007).

### Philosophy and Principles

Osteopathy views the human body in a holistic manner and emphasises an excellent patient–practitioner relationship. It recognises that structure and function of the body are interrelated at all levels (Paulus, 2013). Kuchera and Kuchera (1994) suggest that practitioners of this therapy provide patient care based on the following principles:

- The human body is a unit in which all the parts are interrelated; every individual is a unit of body, mind and spirit.

- The body has its own self-regulatory mechanisms and is capable of self-healing and health maintenance.

- The wellbeing of a person depends on the proper, smooth functioning of all structures in the body, including bones, muscles, tendons, ligaments and organs; the signs and symptoms of a disease or condition arise due to the interplay of multiple physical and nonphysical factors.

In osteopathy, rational treatment is therefore based upon the integration of these principles (Hruby, 2000). This means that by manipulating a patient's bones, muscles and joints, osteopaths tend to aid the body's self-regulatory and self-healing mechanisms, correcting the structural and functional abnormalities.

# Chiropractic

Chiropractic is a form of manual therapy concerned with the diagnosis, treatment and prevention of musculoskeletal disorders. It also helps manage the effects of these disorders on different systems of the body, especially the nervous system (Meeker and Haldeman, 2002). Similarly to osteopaths, chiropractic practitioners use their hands to correct alignment problems, improve function, increase mobility and decrease pain and discomfort in the musculoskeletal system. However, many chiropractors predominantly focus on the problems of the spine, with a specialist interest in back and neck pain (Wardwell, 1992).

## Origin

Daniel David Palmer founded the chiropractic practice as a medical system in 1895. Palmer was born in 1845 in Ontario, Canada, but later migrated to the United States in search of work. In his early life, he held several jobs to make a living. After working for nearly 20 years in a variety of professions, Palmer turned all his efforts towards magnetic healing, a popular therapy of his time. However, the exact details on how he was drawn to becoming a natural healer and learned the techniques of magnetic healing are unclear (Ward, 2015). According to Krieg (1995), he met a famous magnetic healer of the time, named Paul Caster, who later became his teacher on Mesmer's magnetic healing.

Palmer made a 'Great Discovery' on 18 September 1895 when his deaf janitor, Harvey Lillard, did not react to the sound of a noisy fire engine (Wardwell, 1992). Palmer came to know that Lillard's hearing had become severely impaired while lifting a heavy object 17 years earlier. On manual assessment, Palmer discovered a lump in Lillard's back and felt that it might somehow be related to his deafness (Pettman, 2007). Palmer then tried to correct it by giving thrusts on the vertebra; unbelievably, Lillard's hearing was restored. From that time on, the seed of the chiropractic medical system was planted. Two years after the great discovery, Palmer established his first training institute – the Palmer Infirmary and Chiropractic School (now known as the Palmer College of Chiropractic) – in Davenport, Iowa, in 1897 (Baer, 1987).

Shortly thereafter, many students from Europe came to study at this school of chiropractic in order to become chiropractors. The first Europeans to study there are thought to have begun their training in 1906. In the UK, chiropractic was introduced during the early part of the 20th century. Historically, the first Briton to study at the Palmer School was a man from Liverpool named Arthur Eteson (Waddell, 2004). However, unlike osteopathy, the legal recognition of chiropractic as a health profession has been slow. In the UK, the General Chiropractic Council (GCC) was established in 1994, and the professional title 'chiropractor' was not protected by law until 2001 (Keating, Cleveland and Menke, 2004).

**Philosophy and Principles**

Similar to osteopathy, chiropractic has a holistic approach to patient care. It considers the human being as a unit of body, mind and soul, and believes that the body has its own ways to self-heal and self-regulate. However, many chiropractors understand the human being in a more holistic manner than osteopathy. They believe that the human body follows the same laws that govern the universe in general; the overall wellbeing of a person depends on the appropriate balance of the triune of life: intelligence, force and matter. Many chiropractors postulate that a little deviation in these can lead a person to illnesses and other maladies (Haldeman, 2004).

In chiropractic care, the spinal adjustment is usually performed as a core treatment. Chiropractors often focus on the spine and vertebral alignment and extremity joints as the primary means of reducing musculoskeletal pain and discomfort. Many chiropractors believe that misalignment in the spinal column interferes with the travelling of nerve messages between the brain and the rest of the body, which ultimately causes pain and disability in the body (Janse, Houser and Wells, 1947). Thus, by correcting these alignment problems, chiropractors tend to assist the body's self-maintenance mechanisms. Other chiropractors diagnose and treat using a neuromusculoskeletal, biomechanical and anatomical basis, restoring function through the treatment of local structures.

## Similarities between Osteopathy and Chiropractic

Osteopathy and chiropractic practices are similar in many aspects. These include:

- **Origin.** Both practices share a common origin. Their roots can be found in the traditional 'bone setting', and both emerged during the late 19th century in the United States because of the shortcomings in allopathic medicine (Pettman, 2007).

- **Philosophy.** Both practices view the human being in a holistic manner – as a unit of body, mind and soul – and consider the body as an interconnected, functional unit that has the capacity to self-heal and self-regulate (Klein, 1998).

- **Treatment objective.** The primary treatment objective of both these disciplines is the same: reducing bodily aches and pain. Both prioritise the integrity of the spine to ensure the wellbeing of an individual (Vickers and Zollman, 1999).

- **Diagnosis.** Both professions use similar medical history-taking and physical examination processes. Movement palpation (feeling by hand) is predominantly used by both in diagnosing abnormalities of structure (Ward, 2015).

- **Treatment.** Practitioners of both practices use the power of touch in the treatment of their patients. In addition, a significant portion of their workload is very similar. Both primarily work with bones, muscles and connective tissues to treat musculoskeletal pain and disability. In many instances, both use similar techniques to deal with similar conditions (Johnson, Schultz and Ferguson, 1989).

- **Education.** Both professions require a minimum of a degree qualification in the specific discipline in order to practise.

- **Treatment technique.** Spinal manipulation is a treatment technique used by both professions, although the training and application may differ slightly: osteopaths tend to use their limbs to provide levered thrusts, whereas chiropractors are more likely to use their hands, although a crossover between these is common in modern osteopathic and chiropractic training.

- **Treatment duration.** Osteopaths usually treat patients on an 'as needed' basis, whereas chiropractors frequently suggest six sessions to their patients, initially frequent and then at weekly intervals.

As you can see, there are distinct similarities between our professions, but that can be said of all manual therapies and physical therapies. In the modern world, we are less bound by titles and we have started to blend our techniques and skills for the benefit of our patients. This book is not a philosophical discussion, but our contribution to the world of manual therapy, with techniques that we use within our clinical practices on a day-to-day basis.

We hope you enjoy.

*Jimmy, Giles and Ricky*

# References

Baer, H.A. (1987). Divergence and convergence in two systems of manual medicine: Osteopathy and chiropractic in the United States. *Medical Anthropology Quarterly, 1*(2), 176–193.

Haldeman, S. (2004). *Principles and Practice of Chiropractic*. New York, NY: McGraw-Hill Medical.

Hruby, R.J. (2000). *Osteopathic Principles and Philosophy*. Available from https://www.westernu.edu/bin/ime/opp_word.pdf [accessed 18 September 2016].

Janse, J., Houser, R.H. and Wells, B.F. (1947). *Chiropractic Principles and Technic: For Use by Students and Practitioners*. Lombard, IL: National College of Chiropractic.

Johnson, M.R., Schultz, M.K. and Ferguson, A.C. (1989). A comparison of chiropractic, medical and osteopathic care for work-related sprains and strains. *Journal of Manipulative and Physiological Therapeutics, 12*(5), 335–344.

Keating, J.C., Cleveland, C.S. and Menke, M. (2004). *Chiropractic History: A Primer*. Davenport, IA: Association for the History of Chiropractic.

Klein, P. (1998). [Osteopathy and chiropractic]. *Revue medicale de Bruxelles, 19*(4), A283–289.

Krieg, J.C. (1995). Chiropractic manipulation: An historical perspective. *The Iowa Orthopedic Journal, 15*, 95.

Kuchera, W.A. and Kuchera, M.L. (1994). *Osteopathic Principles in Practice*. Dayton, OH: Greyden Press LLC.

Line, O. and Embase, A. (2010). American Osteopathic Association guidelines for osteopathic manipulative treatment (OMT) for patients with low back pain. *Journal of the American Osteopathic Association, 110*(11), 653–666.

Meeker, W.C. and Haldeman, S. (2002). Chiropractic: A profession at the crossroads of mainstream and alternative medicine. *Annals of Internal Medicine, 136*(3), 216–227.

Miller, K. (1998). The evolution of professional identity: The case of osteopathic medicine. *Social Science and Medicine, 47*(11), 1739–1748.

Paulus, S. (2013). The core principles of osteopathic philosophy. *International Journal of Osteopathic Medicine, 16*(1), 11–16.

Pettman, E. (2007). A history of manipulative therapy. *Journal of Manual and Manipulative Therapy, 15*(3), 165–174.

Still, A.T. (1908). *Autobiography of Andrew T. Still*. Kirksville, MO: Author.

Tan, S.Y. and Zia, J.K. (2007). Andrew Taylor Still (1828–1917): Founder of osteopathic medicine. *Singapore Medical Journal, 48*(11), 975.

Vickers, A. and Zollman, C. (1999). ABC of complementary medicine: The manipulative therapies: Osteopathy and chiropractic. *British Medical Journal, 319*(7218), 1176.

Waddell, G. (2004). *The Back Pain Revolution*. Philadelphia, PA: Elsevier Health Sciences.

Ward, C.L. (2015). Osteopathic and chiropractic: An examination of the patient–physician relationship in their respective practices. *Honours Theses*, Paper 403.

Wardwell, W.I. (1992). *Chiropractic: History and Evolution of a New Profession*. Maryland Heights, MO: Mosby-Year Book.

# PART I

# Theory

# CHAPTER 1

# Manipulation Therapy Theory

## Introduction

Manipulation therapy is a type of physical therapy that is practised worldwide by health care professionals in various specialities, such as osteopathy, chiropractic and physiotherapy, to treat musculoskeletal pain and disability (Rubinstein *et al.*, 2011). The therapy uses drug-free, non-surgical techniques to reduce joint pressure, improve joint range of motion, restore muscle and tissue balance, promote body fluid mobilisation, decrease inflammation and enhance nerve function (Di Fabio, 1992; Cyriax, 1973). Scientific research on this modality continues; so far, a number of positive clinical findings have been reported. However, the theoretical base to support every aspect of its therapeutic use is still underdeveloped (Evans, 2010). Hence, the therapy has primarily been used for the management of a range of muscle and joint conditions.

Although the volume of research on joint manipulation has increased significantly in recent years (Bronfort *et al.*, 2008), little is understood about how this therapy works and what physiological effects it causes on various parts of the body (Evans, 2002). To date, many theories have been proposed to interpret these physiological mechanisms, but a unified theory based on scientific evidence is still lacking. However, this chapter is not written to offer a new theory based on the previous literature. Its purpose is to review features suggested to be essential components of manipulation and discuss various theories on physiological mechanisms that have been proposed up to now.

# History

Historically, manipulation is one of the oldest techniques, which has its origins in parallel developments throughout the world (Schiötz and Cyriax, 1975). For thousands of years, it has been widely practised in many cultures to treat a variety of conditions associated with the musculoskeletal and other systems. The techniques have been carried down from one generation to the next (Wiese and Callender, 2005). The earliest record of the practice of spinal manipulation is found in China, which dates back to 2700 BCE (Waddell, 1996). In Europe, Hippocrates (460–385 BCE) was the first physician to describe the manipulation techniques (Withington, 1948).

Despite having an early history of parallel developments in many parts of the world, manipulation therapy has gained and lost favour with the medical profession many times over the centuries (Pettman, 2007). During the renaissance of medicine in the 16th century, Hippocrates' manipulation techniques reappeared in the writings of a number of famous scholars, including Guido Guidi, Johannes Scultetus and Ambrose Paré, as a treatment for musculoskeletal conditions (Anderson, 1983; Pettman, 2007). Nevertheless, by the 18th century, the general acceptance of these techniques was rejected by physicians and surgeons. They viewed manipulation therapy as a practice of folk healers, also known as bonesetters, and attributed its successes more to luck than skill (Lomax, 1975).

From the 19th century onwards, the therapy became an area of dispute among medical professionals. However, because of shortcomings in allopathic medicine and the origination of two leading alternative health care systems, osteopathy and chiropractic, by the end of the 19th century, views about manipulation therapy irrevocably changed (Anderson, 1981); in the early part of the 20th century, medical and osteopathic physicians initially paved the way for introducing manipulation techniques to the physical therapy profession. Since then physical therapists have contributed substantially to the field and solidified manipulation therapy within in its legally regulated scope of practice (Pettman, 2007).

## What is Manipulation?

There is no satisfactory definition of manipulation because of its colloquial function. The term is so vague that many authors have found it very challenging to distinguish 'real' manipulation from its physical therapy counterparts (e.g. Song *et al.*, 2006; Colloca, Keller and Gunzburg, 2004; Harvey *et al.*, 2003). Many researchers have tried to provide a valid definition in diverse sources of literature, but a final definition has not yet been agreed. Moreover, the definition varies across specialities (Maigne and Vautravers, 2003). For example, in osteopathy, manipulation is not regarded as a complete treatment; rather, it is considered a part of the manipulative treatment strategy for a given patient (Wieting and Cugalj, 2008).

In addition, manipulation therapy is different from mobilisation, because, theoretically, it does not allow the recipient to stop joint movement during the procedure, whereas mobilisation techniques involve application of non-thrust passive motion to the spine that can be prevented by the recipient (Corrigan and Maitland, 1983).

In comparing previous definitions and descriptions of manipulation, Evans and Lucas (2010) presented several empirically derived features that are necessary to define 'manipulation' (see box below). The authors divided these features into two categories: the 'action' (that which one person, the practitioner, performs upon another, the patient) and the 'mechanical effect' (that which occurs within the patient, as a result of the action).

## Proposed Empirically Derived Essential Features of Manipulation

**Action (that which the practitioner does to the recipient)**

- A force is applied to the recipient.
- The line of action of this force is perpendicular (at an angle of nearly 90°) to the articular surface of the affected joint.

**Mechanical response (that which occurs within the recipient)**

- The applied force creates motion at a joint.
- This joint motion includes articular surface separation.
- Cavitation occurs within the affected joint.

Source: Evans and Lucas (2010)

# Types of Manipulation

Although there are many disputes about the definition of manipulation, it generally involves a thrust being applied to the recipient through either a long or a short lever-arm (Di Fabio, 1999). Osteopaths developed the long-lever techniques, whereas chiropractors the short-lever techniques (Maigne and Vautravers, 2003).

In *long-lever manipulation* (or low-velocity high-amplitude manipulation), the thrust is delivered in a non-specific manner, not directly to the vertebra – for example, to the shoulder, pelvic region or scapular (Shekelle *et al.*, 1992). During this type of manipulation, the practitioner passively moves many vertebral joints simultaneously within their range of motion (Di Fabio, 1999).

On the other hand, the *short-lever manipulation* (or high-velocity low-amplitude manipulation) involves a low-amplitude thrust being applied at a contact point on a process, such as spinous process, lamina or mammillary process, of a specific lumbar vertebra to affect the vertebral articulation (Bergmann, 2005). During this process, the therapist applies a fast rotational force at an angle of 90° to the overlying skin surface of the affected joint (Cao *et al.*, 2013).

## What is the Cavitation/Crack/Pop?

During high-velocity, low-amplitude (HVLA) manipulation, a strong 'thrust' or 'impulse' is applied perpendicularly to a diarthrodial synovial joint. This action causes separation of the joint surface beyond a certain magnitude, producing an audible cracking sound. The cracking sound often signifies a successful manipulation (Sandoz, 1969), although it has been highly debated whether the sound is an essential feature of the manipulation or not (Brodeur, 1995; Flynn, Childs and Fritz, 2006).

The most widely accepted explanation for the production of this 'crack' sound is an event called 'cavitation', which occurs within the affected joint's synovial fluid (SF) (Evans and Breen, 2006). The term 'cavitation' refers to the formation and activity of gaseous bubbles (or cavities) within the SF of the joint, which are created via local decline in pressure (Evans and Lucas, 2010). Cavitation usually results due to certain types of motion between the articular surfaces and can occur during both high- and low-velocity joint manipulation (Evans and Breen, 2006).

## What is Paraphysiological Space?

Paraphysiological space, also known as a 'zone of end-play' or the 'barrier', is the zone of elasticity between the physiologic barrier and the anatomic barrier (Vernon and Mrozek, 2005). Sandoz (1976) first proposed the presence of a 'paraphysiological space' within the anatomic limit while describing the nature of joint manipulation. The author published a figure (see Figure 1.1) explaining several phases of a joint's total arc of motion during manipulation, and depicted a space beyond the passive range but under the anatomic limit. However, the validity of the Sandoz model has been highly debated in recent years (Symons, Leonard and Herzog, 2002; Ianuzzi and Khalsa, 2005) due to the introduction of a new term 'neutral zone' by spinal biomechanics experts to describe the zone within a joint's motion (Panjabi *et al.*, 1988). As a result, many authors have suggested a revision to the old model (Vernon and Mrozek, 2005).

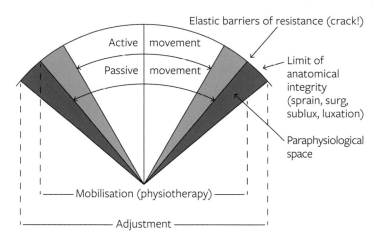

FIGURE 1.1 SANDOZ MODEL

Although some attempts have fallen short of providing a comprehensive revision to the Sandoz model (Gibbons and Tehan, 2001; McCarthy, 2001), Evans and Breen (2006) proposed a new general model of manipulation (see Figure 1.2), considering the requirement of a pre-thrust position and incorporating the 'neutral zone' into the original model. However, future research is required to test this model.

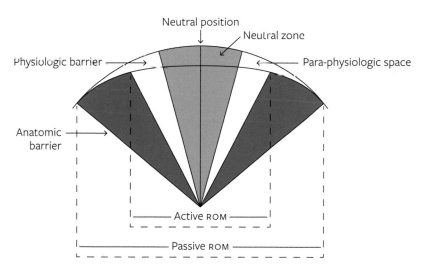

FIGURE 1.2 SCHEMATIC REPRESENTATION OF
THE PROPOSED MODEL BY EVANS AND BREEN (2006)

## Mechanism of Action of Joint Manipulation

Manipulation therapy has some strong clinical evidence for both acute and chronic low back pain (Bronfort *et al.*, 2004; Jüni *et al.*, 2009). However, the mechanism of action behind these clinical effects is only partly understood. Researchers have so far proposed many theories for the possible physiological mechanisms of manipulation, but scientific evidence to support these theories is still limited. This section discusses some of the noteworthy previous and current theories that have been proposed.

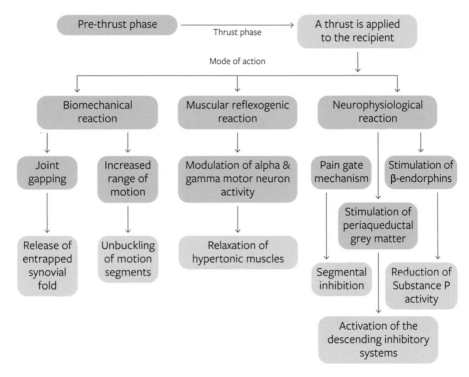

FIGURE 1.3 SCHEMATIC DIAGRAM OF THE PROPOSED PHYSIOLOGICAL MECHANISMS OF SPINAL AND PERIPHERAL MANIPULATION

### Joint Gapping

The theory of joint gapping has a significant importance in understanding the mechanism of joint manipulation. It has been hypothesised that gapping of the facet joint in the spine encourages release of the entrapped meniscoid (Evans, 2002), a capsule process that fills in empty spaces and compensates the incongruence of articular surfaces (Kos, Hert and Sevcik, 2001). Meniscoids are structures that have been thought to play an important role in inducing joint pain, because it has been identified that fibro-adipose meniscoids are capable of creating a painful situation (Bogduk and Jull, 1985; Mercer and Bogduk, 1993). Evans (2002) suggests that a HVLA manipulation, involving the facet joint gapping, results in impaction and an increase in joint space. These changes encourage the meniscoid to go back to its normal anatomic position in the joint cavity; once the meniscoid returns to its position, the joint capsule distension is ceased. As a result, the joint pain is also reduced.

Joint gapping theory is based on the most widely held belief that HVLA manipulation has biomechanical effects. The earliest biomechanical studies (e.g. Roston and Wheeler Haines, 1947; Unsworth, Dowson and Wright, 1971; Sandoz, 1976) to investigate the phenomenon of 'joint cracking' in finger joints (metacarpophalangeal) showed that joint surface separation was associated with the production of an audible 'crack' sound. These studies demonstrated that the separation of joint surfaces resulted in cavitation, the process responsible for the cracking sound, and an immediate increase in radiolucent joint space. Sandoz (1976) reported that this was associated with a 5–10° increase in range of movement at the joint. The author also noted that for about 20 minutes the cracking sound could not be repeated.

Similar results were reported in later biomechanical studies (e.g. Meal and Scott, 1986; Watson, Kernohan and Möllan, 1989) of 'joint cracking' in metacarpophalangeal (MCP) joints. To investigate this phenomenon further, Conway et al. (1993) compared the sounds from the spinal facet joint cavitations with the sounds from the MCP joint distractions. After analysing the sound signals from both the joints, the authors reported similar sound waves and proposed that a similar process was occurring in both joints. This means that HVLA manipulation may also result in an increase in joint space at the facet joints. In a more recent study, Cramer et al. (2000) provided further evidence to support this hypothesis. Using MRI scanning, the authors demonstrated that HVLA thrust caused an immediate increase in joint surface separation. In this study, the average increase in gapping for the HVLA group was +1.2 mm, whereas the average change for the control group was only +0.3 mm.

Although there is a need for further work on a larger group to establish the biomechanical effect of HVLA manipulation, these findings clearly support the hypothesis of joint gapping that manipulation results in a biomechanical separation of the facet joint.

### Unbuckling of Motion Segments

This theory is derived from the oldest concept that spinal manipulation realigns misaligned joints (Hood, 1871). For centuries, there was a long-held belief that traditional practitioners could put the bone back in place by manipulating the joint. This was also the likely reason that manual practitioners earned their name as 'bonesetters' (Bigos, Bowyer and Braen, 1994). Evans (2002) stated that the production of the audible cracking sound and the immediate symptomatic relief following manipulation could be the reasons for the development of this concept.

However, it is now identified that the source behind the 'crack' sound is the phenomenon called cavitation (Evans and Lucas, 2010). Moreover, recent biomechanical studies on the vertebral motion following spinal manipulation have found that the manipulated vertebrae associated with cavitation only show transient relative movements (Gal *et al.*, 1997; Herzog, 2000; Evans 2002). As a result, the old theory of realigning misaligned vertebrae has become an epiphenomenon and a new theory has emerged in its place.

As individual motion segments can buckle, it has been hypothesised that production of relatively large motions at the vertebrae may help attain a new position of stable equilibrium (Wilder, Pope and Frymoyer, 1988). Based on this theory, a variety of hypotheses have been developed over the past decades. Triano (2000) suggested that the mechanical force applied during a high-velocity, low-amplitude thrust (HVLAT) manipulation might deliver enough energy to restore a buckled segment to a lower energy level, thus lessening mechanical stress or strain on soft and hard paraspinal tissues (Pickar, 2002). One of the major reasons behind the developing theory is the long-held hypothesis that spinal manipulation can restore the affected joint mobility and joint play. However, further research into this mechanism is required to establish the theory.

### Reflex Responses

The muscular reflexogenic effect is another important theory that has been thought to play a role in the mechanism of manipulation. The musculature in the human body has some reflex responses, by way of its reflex arcs, to protect itself from potentially harmful force (Evans, 2002). Therefore, when a damaging force is applied to joints, the musculature creates positive synergism between the active (muscular) and passive (capsuloligamentous) joint restraints (Solomonow *et al.*, 1998). This reflexogenic effect is hypothesised to create a reflex mechanism of reducing pain and improving muscle hypertonicity and functional ability (Potter, McCarthy and Oldham, 2005).

Manipulation has long been thought to influence the activation of the musculature through reflex pathways (Wyke, 1979). To confirm this hypothesis, a number of studies have been done over the past decades (e.g. Herzog *et al.*, 1993; Herzog, Scheele and Conway, 1999; Symons *et al.*, 2000; Suter *et al.*, 2005). These studies demonstrated that spinal manipulation caused (excitatory) reflex responses not only in muscles local to the manipulated joint but also in more distant muscles. In addition, in a comparable experiment, Colloca and Keller (2001) measured the electromyographic (EMG) reflex response to spinal manipulation in patients (n – 20) with low back pain. Not surprisingly, the authors reported elicitation of a reflex response in the musculature; however, they also found that those who had frequent to constant pain symptoms had the largest amplitude of reflex response in comparison with those who had infrequent to occasional symptoms.

These studies provide some strong evidence for the fact that spinal manipulation results in reflex muscular contractions through mechanoreceptors in the joint capsules and muscles. However, it is not yet clear whether these reflex responses are actually caused by the joint manipulation, and are not merely artefacts resulting from some other part of the therapy (Potter *et al.*, 2005).

### Modulation of Alpha Motor Neuron Activity

It has long been hypothesised that back pain causes muscle hypertonicity, and that spinal manipulation stimulates nociceptive afferents, which in turn relax or normalise hypertonic muscle through modulating alpha motor neuron activity (Evans, 2002). However, scientific evidence to support this theory is still limited, and there has been some debate on this hypothesis (Potter *et al.*, 2005). The earliest studies done to evaluate this theory suggest that a high-velocity thrust manipulation may activate nociceptive afferents, but only when forces involved with the manipulation are transferred to the surrounding joint capsule and soft tissues (Gillette, 1986, 1987; Herzog *et al.*, 1993). Ahern *et al.* (1988) supported this hypothesis to some extent. The authors reported that a majority of patients with low back pain in their study actually prevented the activation of inhibitory afferents, as they failed to achieve the range of flexion necessary for the relaxation.

Lederman (1997) argued that the activation of inhibitory afferents is highly questionable because sudden stretch produced by high-velocity thrust manipulation would stimulate the motor neuron rather than inhibiting it. In contrast, Dishman and Bulbulian (2000) provided evidence that both spinal manipulation and mobilisation could result in significant but temporary attenuation of alpha motor neuronal excitability. The authors commented that their findings substantiate the theory that spinal manipulation might activate transient inhibitory effects on the human motor system. However, more evidence is needed to establish the theory, as well as its clinical and therapeutic relevance.

**Modulation of Gamma Motor Neuron Activity**

Korr's theory (1975) of the facilitated segment is a decades-old theory that has been used to interpret the mechanism of manipulation. The theory was developed based on outcomes of the early EMG studies (Denslow, 1944; Denslow and Clough, 1941; Denslow, Korr and Krems, 1947). These primitive experiments found that when a stimulus was applied to a painful section, it showed an enhanced EMG response. Recently, Lehman, Vernon and McGill (2001) also demonstrated the same result with a more methodically correct study design. The authors also reported that spinal manipulation seemed to decrease the EMG response to a painful stimulus.

From the early evidential basis, Korr (1975) hypothesised that a painful segment had a facilitatory response, and proposed that an increase in gamma motor neuron activity could lead to muscle hypertonicity by reflexly facilitating the alpha motor neuronal excitability. The author suggested that spinal manipulation could calm the excited gamma motor neurons by increasing joint mobility, producing a barrage of impulses in proprioceptive afferents (muscle spindle and smaller-diameter afferents). However, the neural pathway for this proposed mechanism of spinal manipulation is so far undetermined. Although this mechanism still remains hypothetical, the influence of proprioceptive afferents to the function of the spine and the neurophysiological effects of spinal manipulation on these afferents are gaining increased attention in the scientific community (Pickar, 2002).

However, the theory of the facilitated segment has also raised some debate. Potter *et al.* (2005) suggested that this whole theory is contentious, because it has not yet been proven that patients with back pain have a facilitated alpha motor neuron activity.

## Pain Gate Mechanism

Melzack and Wall's (1967) gate control theory of pain is a revolutionary theory that has been used to explain the modulation of pain perception. The theory proposes that the substantia gelatinosa (SG) layer, which is located in the dorsal horn of the spinal cord, has a gate-like mechanism. Nociceptive (small diameter) A-δ and C sensory fibres carry the pain stimuli to the dorsal horn and 'open' the SG layer, and non-nociceptive (large diameter) A-β fibres (from secondary muscle spindle afferents, joint capsule mechanoreceptor and cutaneous mechanoreceptors) inhibit the transmission of pain signals by A-δ and C fibres and 'close' the layer. In addition, the authors suggested that this mechanism of gate control occurs in the lamina of the dorsal horn, and the mechanism is also influenced by nerve impulses that descend from the brain.

As spinal manipulation can produce a barrage of impulses, it has been thought to modulate the gate-closing mechanism in the dorsal horn through movement of the peri-articular tissues, ultimately stimulating the A-β fibres from muscle spindles and facet joint mechanoreceptors (Potter *et al.*, 2005). However, there is not enough evidence to support this hypothesis; therefore, more work is necessary to establish this theory.

### Descending Inhibitory Mechanism

Descending inhibitory pathways play a significant role in the modulation of pain perception. The periaqueductal grey matter (PAG), a small tube-shaped region of the midbrain, located surrounding the 3rd ventricle serves as the primary control centre for modulating descending pain mechanism. Stimulation of the PAG produces immediate and profound analgesia through the descending PAG pathways (Behbehani, 1995). The dorsal PAG (dPAG) is responsible for sympathoexcitation (processing of fight-or-flight responses, fear and anxiety), whereas the ventral PAG (vPAG) has seemed to be involved in sympatho-inhibition (freezing or disengagement behaviour). Stimulation of the dPAG results a fast-acting, nonopioid-mediated analgesia, and stimulation of the vPAG produces a longer-term, opioid-mediated analgesic response (Satpute *et al.*, 2013).

Activation of the endogenous descending pathways through the dPAG has been thought as a possible mechanism for the antinociceptive effects of HVLA thrust manipulation and as such has gained a considerable amount of attention in the scientific community (Thomson, Haig and Mansfield, 2009). In support of this theory, a large body of literature has already suggested that hypoalgesic and sympathoexcitatory effects following spinal manipulation could be a result of the activation of descending inhibitory systems (Wright, 1995; Vicenzino, Collins and Wright, 1996; Vernon, 2000; Potter *et al.*, 2005). The relationship between these effects has also been studied. In their investigation on the possible correlation between spinal manipulation-induced hypoalgesia and sympathoexcitation, Vincenzino, Collins and Wright (1998) found that there was a strong interrelation between the two effects, and suggested that this might be due to the activation of a central control mechanism.

### Neurotransmitters

Several neurotransmitters have been identified as potential brain chemicals that are involved in the modulation of pain perception. Substance P (SP), an 11-amino acid polypeptide, is one of the widely studied neurotransmitters, which assists in the central transmission of nociceptive input (Kandel, Schwartz and Jessell, 2000). SP is produced in the dorsal root ganglion (DRG) and has been shown to modulate pain processing, neurogenic inflammation and spinal reflex activity. It is released into the peripheral tissues and dorsal horn of the spinal cord by unmyelinated C-polymodal nociceptors (Nyberg, Sharma and Wiesenfeld-Hallin, 1995).

It has been hypothesised that β-endorphins, which are derived from pituitary gland secretion, activate the endogenous antinociceptive system by reducing the activity of SP in the dorsal horn, thereby blocking the transmission of afferent nociceptive input to the higher centres of the brain (Kandel *et al.*, 2000; Potter *et al.*, 2005). Based on this hypothesis, a number of studies have suggested that the hypoalgesic effect seen following spinal manipulation is due to the antinociceptive influence of β-endorphins (Thomson *et al.*, 2009). Vernon *et al.* (1986) studied this theory on a small group of subjects (n = 21) by assessing their plasma β-endorphin levels following the intervention. The authors demonstrated that the HVLAT group showed a significant increase in β-endorphins levels compared with the group that received a sham manipulation. Unfortunately, later studies on the release of β-endorphins by spinal manipulation have so far failed to display any significant effect (Christian *et al.*, 1988; Sanders *et al.*, 1990). Moreover, these studies reported no substantial variance between the experimental and control group in the release of β-endorphins. However, Vernon (2000) and Wright (1995) have highlighted that there were methodological flaws in those experiments – for example, the assay had low sensitivity to detect baseline β-endorphin levels.

## Physiological Effects of Manipulation

Manipulation is one of the oldest techniques that is still in use today. However, little is known about the physiological effects of manipulation by which it may provide its therapeutic benefit. This section reviews the current theories on the effects of manipulation that have been proposed to date.

### Effects on the Vertebral Bodies

At a very basic level, manipulation involves a thrust (or an external force) being applied to the patient. The thrust is introduced either to a chosen vertebral motion segment or to a part of the body that serves as a lever (Maigne and Vautravers, 2003). The paraspinal soft tissues absorb a majority of the thrust and the spine absorbs the rest (Triano, 1992), mobilising the vertebrae on one another. The mobilisation of the vertebrae following manipulation has been established in cadaver studies. Gal *et al.* (1997) used high-speed cinematography to record the movements; using needles threaded into the thoracic vertebrae (T10, T11 and T12), the authors showed that there were substantial relative movements between the targeted and immediately adjacent vertebrae following the thrusts. In another study on the relative movement of the lumbar vertebrae following spinal manipulation, Maigne and Guillon (2000) used monoaxial accelerometers to demonstrate that there were relative intervertebral movements during the thrust.

However, the produced movement at the vertebral level during spinal manipulation is complex, because manipulation applies non-physiological forces and several adjacent levels are mobilised simultaneously. Taken together, it can be said that manipulation results in vertebral movements not only at the target segment but also at the adjacent levels, and the induced movement occurs in combination.

### Effects on the Facet Joints

The physiological effects on the facet joints by HVLAT manipulation have been suggested to be force threshold-dependent (Triano, Brennan and McGregor, 1991; Evans, 2002). In the thoracic spine, the threshold was found between 450N and 500N; in the lumbar spine, the threshold was 400N (Brennan, 1995).

The articular surfaces of the facet joints do not separate in the course of physiological rotation (McFadden and Taylor, 1990). The separation does not happen even if the thrust is applied. After the thrust is introduced to the facet joint, the articular surfaces keep adhering with each other and the vertebrae remain inter-reliant (Maigne and Vautravers, 2003). However, when the thrust force goes beyond the threshold, separation of the surfaces takes place suddenly, with an audible 'click' or 'crack' sound. As a result, cavitation occurs within the SF of the affected joint (Evans and Lucas, 2010).

### Effects on the Intervertebral Discs

Spinal manipulation has a physiological effect on the intervertebral discs. Maigne and Guillon (2000) used accelerometers to demonstrate that manipulation could produce transient but significant change in intradiscal pressure. To measure this pressure in the lumbar spine, the authors used two different side-posture manipulation techniques. However, the techniques varied only in the sagittal plane position. The authors found that there was a small initial increase in intradiscal pressure when the thrust was introduced; at the end of the thrust, this was speedily followed by a decrease in pressure below the baseline value. The authors also found that the change in pressure correlated with the intervertebral movement. This finding means that intradiscal pressure corresponds to the changes in the spinal segment.

The findings of this study are consistent with some of the earliest theories that have been used to explain disc-related back-pain problems. One important theory is that manipulation allows protruding disc material to return to its central position by decreasing the intradiscal pressure (Maigne and Nieves, 2005; d'Ornano *et al.*, 1990). However, no studies have so far demonstrated gross reductions in herniation size after manipulation (Maigne and Vautravers, 2003). Another theory is that manipulation allows repositioning of the joint by separating the articular surfaces and diminishing the intradiscal pressure, which eventually restore the pressure balance throughout the disc (Oliphant, 2004). This theory is more convincing than the mechanism by Maigne and Guillon (2000), because an early observational study by Adams *et al.* (1996) found that diseased discs caused localised pressure peaks corresponding to the areas of high stress concentration. However, further in vivo studies are required.

**Effects on the Paraspinal Muscles**

It has long been thought that manipulation has distinct physiological effects on the paraspinal muscles, as it has been demonstrated in various studies that when a muscle is tapped or stretched, it leads to a pattern of events (Potter *et al.*, 2005). In addition, the mechanical force introduced into a vertebral segment following manipulation has shown to either excite or quiet non-nociceptive, mechanosensitive receptive nerve endings in paraspinal tissues, including facet joints, muscle and intervertebral disc (Pickar, 2002). Although the origin of these responses has been subjected to some debate, it can be said that manipulation definitely has some effect on the paraspinal muscles.

In general, long-lever manipulation has been shown to produce more marked stretching of the paraspinal muscles than short-lever manipulation. For example, the loading phase of the long-lever techniques stretches the paraspinal muscles and psoas on one side and relaxes them on the other side. When the mechanical thrust is applied, intervertebral movement and separation of the facet joints occur; these changes further increase the stretch. Maigne and Vautravers (2003) hypothesised that this increase in stretch might relax the paraspinal muscles by modulating motor neuron activity, particularly alpha and gamma motor neurons.

### Effect on Blood Flow

In traditional osteopathy, one of the goals of manipulation is to improve the blood flow to organs. It has been thought that increase in blood flow might encourage clearance of toxic substances from the body, thus proving to be of benefit in many diseases and conditions (Maigne and Vautravers, 2003). However, there is so far no statistically significant evidence that manipulation increases arterial blood flow or that an increase in vertebral artery flow could be beneficial. In a randomised, controlled and observer-blinded study, Licht *et al.* (1997) observed that there was no change in peak flow velocity following manipulation. Furthermore, in a more recent study, Stelle *et al.* (2014) also could not confirm this hypothesis due to lack of statistical significance, but there was a slight increase in blood flow of vertebral, intracranial and basilar arteries following manipulation.

### Placebo Effect

There have been some debates about whether the physiological effects of manipulation are purely a placebo or more than a placebo. Although the critics of manipulation therapy still regard its successes as a complete placebo effect, a large proportion of the studies have demonstrated a hypoalgesic effect that is significantly different from placebo (Vernon *et al.*, 1990; Vicenzino *et al.*, 1996; Fryer, Carub and McIver, 2004; Thomson *et al.*, 2009). Moreover, the biomechanical effects of manipulation have been widely accepted in much of the literature (Evans and Breen, 2006; Herzog, 2010).

Taken together, it can be said that, as with all interventions, there is likely to be a placebo effect with manipulation. Although the physiological mechanisms of manipulation are still a mystery, it has indeed been demonstrated that this therapy has a substantial psychological effect. It has been identified that the feeling of returning the misaligned joint back to its normal place, the production of the audible cracking sound and the manual contact during the preload and loading phases all contributes to a significant placebo effect (Maigne and Vautravers, 2003). In addition, the immediate symptomatic relief of pain following the manipulation also plays a strong role in inducing a positive psychological effect. Therefore, if the patient and practitioner are benefiting from applying the manipulation techniques in clinical practice, the placebo effects should not be underrated and must be considered as a valid element, as long as no potential risk arises from the intervention (Potter *et al.*, 2005).

## Safety of Manipulation Therapy

In general, manipulation is safe for the treatment of musculoskeletal conditions, when it is administered correctly. The primary adverse issues include temporary exacerbation of symptoms or new local symptoms. Serious complications of manipulation are rarely reported (Triano, 2001). However, cervical spine manipulation has been found to be associated with some serious risks, including stroke, vascular accidents and non-vascular complications (Puentedura *et al.*, 2012). As a result, many researchers have expressed doubt about the safety of this modality and commented that risks associated with the procedures may offset the benefits (Di Fabio, 1999; Ernst, 2007).

The debate regarding the safety of cervical spine manipulation is not a new one. It has been a safety concern since the first adverse event was reported back in 1907 (Rivett, 2006). Although many of these concerns have come from epidemiologic inference, there has been little agreement between incidence reports of adverse events (Puentedura *et al.*, 2012). Estimates of the risk have been reported to vary from 1:50,000 to 1:5.85 million (Haldeman *et al.*, 2001; Magarey *et al.*, 2004). These data clearly suggest that the risks associated with upper spinal manipulation are very low, as millions of cervical manipulations are performed without adverse effects.

Nevertheless, the risk of vascular accident is not negligible, because the common adverse effect reported in most studies is vertebral artery dissection, which has been thought to result due to over-stretching of the artery during rotational manipulation (Nadgir *et al.*, 2003). The majority of these incidents have occurred at the level of the atlantoaxial joint and involved the vertebrobasilar system, particularly the distal loop of the vertebral artery (Haldeman, Kohlbeck and McGregor, 1999). Consequently, it has been hypothesised that cervical spine manipulation may cause stretch-induced damage to the vertebral artery (Herzog, 2010).

In contrast, Symons *et al.* (2002) and Herzog and Symons (2002) demonstrated that stretches to the vertebral artery produced during cervical spine manipulation were much smaller than those that were produced during normal everyday movements. The authors also reported that the elongations produced following spinal manipulations did not induce any tensile forces in the vertebral artery, thus suggesting that spinal manipulation is harmless (Herzog, 2010). In addition, when the experimental neck loads from spinal manipulation were compared with the moment loads tolerated by human volunteers, it was found that sudden neck moments tolerated by volunteers were greater than those observed during the manipulation of the neck (Triano, 2001). In light of the above evidence, it can be said that little is known so far about the transmission of stresses and sudden moment loads across the neck following cervical spine manipulation; therefore, more research is needed.

Although there have been some differences in views regarding adverse events following cervical spine manipulation, Refshauge *et al.* (2002) speculated that these incidents are predictable and might be attributed to inadequate examination and judgement by the practitioner as well as poor skill or incorrect use of techniques. Therefore, it has been suggested that special caution should be taken while performing first-line cervical manipulation.

## Conclusion

From the above discussion, it can be concluded that manipulation is a vast field of investigation and its physiological mechanisms yet understood are overly complex. In addition, there seem to be three different modes of action of manipulation: biomechanical, muscular reflexogenic and neurophysiological mechanisms. However, further insights are needed to have a complete understanding of the basic mechanism of manipulation. Studies researching its neurophysiological and biomechanical mechanisms should therefore develop and apply adequate experimental approaches to better explore the mechanisms. Moreover, as there is no theoretical framework to comprehend the physiological effects of manipulation, it is essential that this area has more high-quality research, particularly in vivo studies on cervical and thoracic manipulation, in order to understand how manipulation provides its reported therapeutic benefits.

## References

Adams, M.A., McMillan, D.W., Green, T.P. and Dolan, P. (1996). Sustained loading generates stress concentrations in lumbar intervertebral discs. *Spine, 21*(4), 434–438.

Ahern, D.K., Follick, M.J., Council, J.R., Laser-Wolston, N. and Litchman, H. (1988). Comparison of lumbar paravertebral EMG patterns in chronic low back pain patients and non-patient controls. *Pain, 34*(2), 153–160.

Anderson, R. (1981). Wharton Hood, MD, the rejected father of manual medicine. *Archives of the California Chiropractic Association, 5*(2), 59–63.

Anderson, R.T. (1983). On doctors and bonesetters in the 16th and 17th centuries. *Chiropractic History: The Archives and Journal of the Association for the History of Chiropractic, 3*(1), 11.

Behbehani, M.M. (1995). Functional characteristics of the midbrain periaqueductal gray. *Progress in Neurobiology, 46*(6), 575–605.

Bergmann, T.F. (2005). High-velocity low-amplitude manipulative techniques. In S. Haldeman (Ed.), *Principles and Practice of Chiropractic*, 3rd edition. McGraw-Hill, 755–766.

Bigos, S.J., Bowyer, O. and Braen, G. (1994). *Acute Low Back Problems in Adults*. Rockville, MD: US Dept. of Health and Human Services. Public Health Service, Agency for Health Care Policy and Research.

Bogduk, N. and Jull, G. (1985). The theoretical pathology of acute locked back: A basis for manipulative therapy. *Manual Medicine, 1*(78), 67.

Brennan, P.C. (1995). Review of the systemic effects of spinal manipulation. In M.I. Gatterman (Ed.), *Foundations of Chiropractic: Subluxation*. St Louis, MO: Elsevier Mosby.

Brodeur, R. (1995). The audible release associated with joint manipulation. *Journal of Manipulative and Physiological Therapeutics, 18,* 155–164.

Bronfort, G., Haas, M., Evans, R.L. and Bouter, L.M. (2004). Efficacy of spinal manipulation and mobilization for low back pain and neck pain: A systematic review and best evidence synthesis. *The Spine Journal, 4*(3), 335–356.

Bronfort, G., Haas, M., Evans, R., Kawchuk, G. and Dagenais, S. (2008). Evidence-informed management of chronic low back pain with spinal manipulation and mobilization. *The Spine Journal, 8*(1), 213–225.

Cao, D.Y., Reed, W.R., Long, C.R., Kawchuk, G.N. and Pickar, J.G. (2013). Effects of thrust amplitude and duration of high-velocity, low-amplitude spinal manipulation on lumbar muscle spindle responses to vertebral position and movement. *Journal of Manipulative and Physiological Therapeutics, 36*(2), 68–77.

Christian, G.F., Stanton, G.J., Sissons, D., How, H.Y. *et al.* (1988). Immunoreactive ACTH, [beta]-endorphin, and cortisol levels in plasma following spinal manipulative therapy. *Spine, 13*(12), 1411–1417.

Colloca, C.J. and Keller, T.S. (2001). Electromyographic reflex responses to mechanical force, manually assisted spinal manipulative therapy. *Spine, 26*(10), 1117–1124.

Colloca, C.J., Keller, T.S. and Gunzburg, R. (2004). Biomechanical and neurophysiological responses to spinal manipulation in patients with lumbar radiculopathy. *Journal of Manipulative and Physiological Therapeutics, 27*(1), 1–15.

Conway, P.J.W., Herzog, W., Zhang, Y., Hasler, E.M. and Ladly, K. (1993). Forces required to cause cavitation during spinal manipulation of the thoracic spine. *Clinical Biomechanics, 8*(4), 210–214.

Corrigan, B. and Maitland, G.D. (1983). *Practical Orthopaedic Medicine.* Butterworth-Heinemann.

Cramer, G.D., Tuck, N.R., Knudsen, J.T., Fonda, S.D. *et al.* (2000). Effects of side-posture positioning and side-posture adjusting on the lumbar zygapophysial joints as evaluated by magnetic resonance imaging: A before and after study with randomization. *Journal of Manipulative and Physiological Therapeutics, 23*(6), 380–394.

Cyriax, J. (1973). Textbook of orthopaedic medicine, Volume II, Treatment by manipulation, massage and injection. *American Journal of Physical Medicine and Rehabilitation, 52*(1), 46.

Denslow, J.S. (1944). An analysis of the variability of spinal reflex thresholds. *Journal of Neurophysiology, 7*(4), 207–215.

Denslow, J.S. and Clough, G.H. (1941). Reflex activity in the spinal extensors. *Journal of Neurophysiology, 4*(6), 430–437.

Denslow, J.S., Korr, I.M. and Krems, A.D. (1947). Quantitative studies of chronic facilitation in human motoneuron pools. *American Journal of Physiology – Legacy Content, 150*(2), 229–238.

Di Fabio, R.P. (1992). Efficacy of manual therapy. *Physical Therapy, 72*(12), 853–864.

Di Fabio, R.P. (1999). Manipulation of the cervical spine: Risks and benefits. *Physical Therapy, 79*(1), 50–65.

Dishman, J.D. and Bulbulian, R. (2000). Spinal reflex attenuation associated with spinal manipulation. *Spine, 25*(19), 2519–2525.

d'Ornano, J., Conrozier, T., Bossard, D., Bochu, M. and Vignon, E. (1990). Effets des manipulations vertebrales sur la hernie discale lombaire. *La Revue de médecine orthopédique, 19*, 21–25.

Ernst, E. (2007). Adverse effects of spinal manipulation: A systematic review. *Journal of the Royal Society of Medicine, 100*(7), 330–338.

Evans, D.W. (2002). Mechanisms and effects of spinal high-velocity, low-amplitude thrust manipulation: Previous theories. *Journal of Manipulative and Physiological Therapeutics, 25*(4), 251–262.

Evans, D.W. (2010). Why do spinal manipulation techniques take the form they do? Towards a general model of spinal manipulation. *Manual Therapy, 15*(3), 212–219.

Evans, D.W. and Breen, A.C. (2006). A biomechanical model for mechanically efficient cavitation production during spinal manipulation: Prethrust position and the neutral zone. *Journal of Manipulative and Physiological Therapeutics, 29*(1), 72–82.

Evans, D.W. and Lucas, N. (2010). What is 'manipulation'? A reappraisal. *Manual Therapy, 15*(3), 286–291.

Flynn, T.W., Childs, J.D. and Fritz, J.M. (2006). The audible pop from high-velocity thrust manipulation and outcome in individuals with low back pain. *Journal of Manipulative and Physiological Therapeutics, 29*(1), 40–45.

Fryer, G., Carub, J. and McIver, S. (2004). The effect of manipulation and mobilisation on pressure pain thresholds in the thoracic spine. *Journal of Osteopathic Medicine, 7*(1), 8–14.

Gal, J., Herzog, W., Kawchuk, G., Conway, P.J. and Zhang, Y.T. (1997). Movements of vertebrae during manipulative thrusts to unembalmed human cadavers. *Journal of Manipulative and Physiological Therapeutics, 20*(1), 30–40.

Gibbons, P. and Tehan, P. (2001). Patient positioning and spinal locking for lumbar spine rotation manipulation. *Manual Therapy, 6*(3), 130–138.

Gillette, R.G. (1986). Potential antinociceptive effects of high-level somatic stimulation: Chiropractic manipulation therapy may coactivate both tonic and phasic analgesic systems. Some recent neurophysiological evidence. *Trans Pac Consortium Res, 1*, A4.

Gillette, R.G. (1987). A speculative argument for the coactivation of diverse somatic receptor populations by forceful chiropractic adjustments. *Manual Medicine, 3*, 1–14.

Haldeman, S., Carey, P., Townsend, M. and Papadopoulos, C. (2001). Arterial dissections following cervical manipulation: The chiropractic experience. *Canadian Medical Association Journal, 165*(7), 905–906.

Haldeman, S., Kohlbeck, F.J. and McGregor, M. (1999). Risk factors and precipitating neck movements causing vertebrobasilar artery dissection after cervical trauma and spinal manipulation. *Spine, 24*(8), 785–794.

Harvey, E., Burton, A.K., Moffett, J.K., Breen, A. and UK BEAM trial team. (2003). Spinal manipulation for low-back pain: A treatment package agreed by the UK chiropractic, osteopathy and physiotherapy professional associations. *Manual Therapy, 8*(1), 46–51.

Herzog, W. (2000). The mechanical, neuromuscular, and physiologic effects produced by spinal manipulation. In: *Clinical Biomechanics of Spinal Manipulation*. Churchill Livingstone.

Herzog, W. (2010). The biomechanics of spinal manipulation. *Journal of Bodywork and Movement Therapies, 14*(3), 280–286.

Herzog, W. and Symons, B. (2002). The mechanics of neck manipulation with special consideration of the vertebral artery. *The Journal of the Canadian Chiropractic Association, 46*(3), 134.

Herzog, W., Conway, P.J., Kawchuk, G.N., Zhang, Y. and Hasler, E.M. (1993). Forces exerted during spinal manipulative therapy. *Spine, 18*(9), 1206–1212.

Herzog, W., Scheele, D. and Conway, P.J. (1999). Electromyographic responses of back and limb muscles associated with spinal manipulative therapy. *Spine, 24*(2), 146–152.

Herzog, W., Zhang, Y.T., Conway, P.J. and Kawchuk, G.N. (1993). Cavitation sounds during spinal manipulative treatments. *Journal of Manipulative and Physiological Therapeutics, 16*(8), 523–526.

Hood, W. (1871). On the so-called 'bone-setting', its nature and results. *The Lancet, 97*(2481), 372–374.

Ianuzzi, A. and Khalsa, P.S. (2005). Comparison of human lumbar facet joint capsule strains during simulated high-velocity, low-amplitude spinal manipulation versus physiological motions. *The Spine Journal, 5*(3), 277–290.

Jüni, P., Battaglia, M., Nüesch, E., Hämmerle, G. *et al.* (2009). A randomised controlled trial of spinal manipulative therapy in acute low back pain. *Annals of the Rheumatic Diseases, 68*(9), 1420–1427.

Kandel, E.R., Schwartz, J.H. and Jessell, T.M. (Eds) (2000). *Principles of Neural Science*, Vol. 4. New York, NY: McGraw-Hill.

Korr, I. M. (1975). Proprioceptors and somatic dysfunction. *Journal of the American Osteopathic Association, 74*(7), 638–650.

Kos, J., Hert, J. and Sevcik, P. (2001). [Meniscoids of the intervertebral joints]. *Acta chirurgiae orthopaedicae et traumatologiae Cechoslovaca, 69*(3), 149–157.

Lederman, E. (1997). *Fundamentals of Manual Therapy: Physiology, Neurology, and Psychology*. Churchill Livingstone.

Lehman, G.J., Vernon, H. and McGill, S.M. (2001). Effects of a mechanical pain stimulus on erector spinae activity before and after a spinal manipulation in patients with back pain: A preliminary investigation. *Journal of Manipulative and Physiological Therapeutics, 24*(6), 402–406.

Licht, P.B., Christensen, H.W., Højgaard, P. and Marving, J. (1997). Vertebral artery flow and spinal manipulation: A randomized, controlled and observer-blinded study. *Journal of Manipulative and Physiological Therapeutics, 21*(3), 141–144.

Lomax, E. (1975). *Manipulative Therapy: A Historical Perspective from Ancient Times to the Modern Era. The Research Status of Spinal Manipulative Therapy*. Washington, DC: US Government Printing Office.

Magarey, M.E., Rebbeck, T., Coughlan, B., Grimmer, K., Rivett, D.A. and Refshauge, K. (2004). Pre-manipulative testing of the cervical spine review, revision and new clinical guidelines. *Manual Therapy, 9*(2), 95–108.

Maigne, J.Y. and Guillon, F. (2000). Highlighting of intervertebral movements and variations of intradiskal pressure during lumbar spine manipulation: A feasibility study. *Journal of Manipulative and Physiological Therapeutics, 23*(8), 531–535.

Maigne, J.Y. and Vautravers, P. (2003). Mechanism of action of spinal manipulative therapy. *Joint Bone Spine, 70*(5), 336–341.

Maigne, R. and Nieves, W.L. (2005). *Diagnosis and Treatment of Pain of Vertebral Origin* (Vol. 1). Boca Raton, FL: Taylor & Francis.

McCarthy, C.J. (2001). Spinal manipulative thrust technique using combined movement theory. *Manual Therapy, 6*(4), 197–204.

McFadden, K.D. and Taylor, J.R. (1990). Axial rotation in the lumbar spine and gaping of the zygapophyseal joints. *Spine, 15*(4), 295–299.

Meal, G.M. and Scott, R.A. (1986). Analysis of the joint crack by simultaneous recording of sound and tension. *Journal of Manipulative and Physiological Therapeutics, 9*(3), 189–195.

Melzack, R. and Wall, P.D. (1967). Pain mechanisms: A new theory. *Survey of Anesthesiology, 11*(2), 89–90.

Mercer, S. and Bogduk, N. (1993). Intra-articular inclusions of the cervical synovial joints. *Rheumatology, 32*(8), 705–710.

Nadgir, R.N., Loevner, L.A., Ahmed, T., Moonis, G. *et al.* (2003). Simultaneous bilateral internal carotid and vertebral artery dissection following chiropractic manipulation: Case report and review of the literature. *Neuroradiology, 45*(5), 311–314.

Nyberg, F., Sharma, H.S. and Wiesenfeld-Hallin, Z. (1995). Neuropeptides and spinal cord reflexes. *Neuropeptides in the Spinal Cord, 104*, 271.

Oliphant, D. (2004). Safety of spinal manipulation in the treatment of lumbar disk herniations: A systematic review and risk assessment. *Journal of Manipulative and Physiological Therapeutics, 27*(3), 197–210.

Panjabi, M., Dvorak, J., Duranceau, J., Yamamoto, I., Gerber, M., Rauschning, W. and Bueff, H. U. (1988). Three-dimensional movements of the upper cervical spine. *Spine, 13*(7), 726–730.

Pettman, E. (2007). A history of manipulative therapy. *Journal of Manual and Manipulative Therapy, 15*(3), 165–174.

Pickar, J.G. (2002). Neurophysiological effects of spinal manipulation. *The Spine Journal, 2*(5), 357–371.

Potter, L., McCarthy, C. and Oldham, J. (2005). Physiological effects of spinal manipulation: A review of proposed theories. *Physical Therapy Reviews, 10*(3), 163–170.

Puentedura, E.J., March, J., Anders, J., Perez, A. *et al.* (2012). Safety of cervical spine manipulation: Are adverse events preventable and are manipulations being performed appropriately? A review of 134 case reports. *Journal of Manual and Manipulative Therapy, 20*(2), 66–74.

Refshauge, K.M., Parry, S., Shirley, D., Larsen, D., Rivett, D.A. and Boland, R. (2002). Professional responsibility in relation to cervical spine manipulation. *Australian Journal of Physiotherapy, 48*(3), 171–179.

Rivett, D.A. (2006). Adverse events and the vertebral artery: Can they be averted? *Manual Therapy, 11*(4), 241–242.

Roston, J.B. and Wheeler Haines, R. (1947). Cracking in the metacarpo-phalangeal joint. *Journal of Anatomy, 81*(2), 165.

Rubinstein, S.M., van Middelkoop, M., Assendelft, W. J., de Boer, M.R. and van Tulder, M.W. (2011). Spinal manipulative therapy for chronic low-back pain. *Cochrane Database of Systematic Reviews, 16*(2).

Sanders, G.E., Reinert, O., Tepe, R. and Maloney, P. (1990). Chiropractic adjustive manipulation on subjects with acute low back pain: Visual analog pain scores and plasma beta-endorphin levels. *Journal of Manipulative and Physiological Therapeutics, 13*(7), 391–395.

Sandoz, R. (1969). The significance of the manipulative crack and of other articular noises. *Annals of the Swiss Chiropractic Association, 4*, 47–68.

Sandoz, R. (1976). Some physical mechanisms and effects of spinal adjustments. *Annals of the Swiss Chiropractic Association, 6*(2), 91–142.

Satpute, A.B., Wager, T.D., Cohen-Adad, J., Bianciardi, M. *et al.* (2013). Identification of discrete functional subregions of the human periaqueductal gray. *Proceedings of the National Academy of Sciences, 110*(42), 17101–17106.

Schiötz, E.H. and Cyriax, J. H. (1975). *Manipulation Past and Present: With an Extensive Bibliography*. London: Heinemann Medical.

Shekelle, P.G., Adams, A.H., Chassin, M.R., Hurwitz, E.L. and Brook, R.H. (1992). Spinal manipulation for low-back pain. *Annals of Internal Medicine, 117*(7), 590–598.

Solomonow, M., Zhou, B.H., Harris, M., Lu, Y. and Baratta, R.V. (1998). The ligamento-muscular stabilizing system of the spine. *Spine, 23*(23), 2552–2562.

Song, X.J., Gan, Q., Cao, J.L., Wang, Z.B. and Rupert, R.L. (2006). Spinal manipulation reduces pain and hyperalgesia after lumbar intervertebral foramen inflammation in the rat. *Journal of Manipulative and Physiological Therapeutics, 29*(1), 5–13.

Stelle, R., Zeigelboim, B.S., Lange, M.C. and Marques, J.M. (2014). Influence of osteopathic manipulation on blood flow velocity of the cerebral circulation in chronic mechanical neck pain. *Revista Dor, 15*(4), 281–286.

Suter, E., Herzog, W., Conway, P.J. and Zhang, Y.T. (2005). Reflex response associated with manipulative treatment of the thoracic spine. *Manuelle Medizin, 43*(5), 305–310.

Symons, B.P., Herzog, W., Leonard, T. and Nguyen, H. (2000). Reflex responses associated with activator treatment. *Journal of Manipulative and Physiological Therapeutics, 23*(3), 155–159.

Symons, B.P., Leonard, T. and Herzog, W. (2002). Internal forces sustained by the vertebral artery during spinal manipulative therapy. *Journal of Manipulative and Physiological Therapeutics, 25*(8), 504–510.

Thomson, O., Haig, L. and Mansfield, H. (2009). The effects of high-velocity low-amplitude thrust manipulation and mobilisation techniques on pressure pain threshold in the lumbar spine. *International Journal of Osteopathic Medicine, 12*(2), 56–62.

Triano, J. (2000). The mechanics of spinal manipulation. In W. Herzog (Ed.), *Clinical Biomechanics of Spinal Manipulation*. Churchill Livingstone, 92–190.

Triano, J.J. (1992). Studies on the biomechanical effect of a spinal adjustment. *Journal of Manipulative and Physiological Therapeutics, 15*(1), 71.

Triano, J.J. (2001). Biomechanics of spinal manipulative therapy. *The Spine Journal, 1*(2), 121–130.

Triano, J.J., Brennan, P.C. and McGregor, M. (1991). A study of threshold response to thoracic manipulation. In: *Proceedings of the 1991 International Conference on Spinal Manipulation*, Arlington, Virginia.

Unsworth, A., Dowson, D. and Wright, V. (1971). 'Cracking joints': A bioengineering study of cavitation in the metacarpophalangeal joint. *Annals of the Rheumatic Diseases, 30*(4), 348.

Vernon, H. (2000). Qualitative review of studies of manipulation-induced hypoalgesia. *Journal of Manipulative and Physiological Therapeutics, 23*(2), 134–138.

Vernon, H.T., Aker, P., Burns, S., Viljakaanen, S. and Short, L. (1990). Pressure pain threshold evaluation of the effect of spinal manipulation in the treatment of chronic neck pain: A pilot study. *Journal of Manipulative and Physiological Therapeutics, 13*(1), 13–16.

Vernon, H.T., Dhami, M.S., Howley, T.P. and Annett, R. (1986). Spinal manipulation and beta-endorphin: A controlled study of the effect of a spinal manipulation on plasma beta-endorphin levels in normal males. *Journal of Manipulative and Physiological Therapeutics, 9*(2), 115–123.

Vernon, H. and Mrozek, J. (2005). A revised definition of manipulation. *Journal of Manipulative and Physiological Therapeutics, 28*(1), 68–72.

Vicenzino, B., Collins, D. and Wright, A. (1996). The initial effects of a cervical spine manipulative physiotherapy treatment on the pain and dysfunction of lateral epicondylalgia. *Pain, 68*(1), 69–74.

Vincenzino, B., Collins, D. and Wright, A. (1998). An investigation of the interrelationship between manipulative therapy-induced hypoalgesia and sympathoexcitation. *Journal of Manipulative Physiology Therapeutics, 21*(7), 448–453.

Waddell, G. (1996). Low back pain: A twentieth century health care enigma. *Spine, 21*(24), 2820–2825.

Watson, P., Kernohan, W.G. and Möllan, R.A.B. (1989). A study of the cracking sounds from the metacarpophalangeal joint. *Proceedings of the Institution of Mechanical Engineers, Part H: Journal of Engineering in Medicine, 203*(2), 109–118.

Wiese, G. and Callender, A. (2005). *History of Spinal Manipulation: Principles and Practice of Chiropractic*, 3rd edition. New York: McGraw-Hill.

Wieting, J.M. and Cugalj, A.P. (2008). Massage, traction, and manipulation. eMedicine. Available at http://emedicine.medscape.com/article/324694-overview (accessed 18 December 2016).

Wilder, D.G., Pope, M.H. and Frymoyer, J.W. (1988). The biomechanics of lumbar disc herniation and the effect of overload and instability. *Journal of Spinal Disorders and Techniques, 1*(1), 16–32.

Withington, E.T. (1948). *Hippocrates: With an English Translation*. Cambridge, MA: Harvard University Press.

Wright, A. (1995). Hypoalgesia post-manipulative therapy: A review of a potential neurophysiological mechanism. *Manual Therapy, 1*(1), 11–16.

Wyke, B. (1979). Neurology of the cervical spinal joints. *Physiotherapy, 65*(3), 72.

# CHAPTER 2

# The Neurophysiology of Manipulation

## Central Effects

Manipulation has been reported to cause numerous neurophysiological effects at both the spinal cord and cortical levels. One of the proposed central effects is called facilitation or sensitisation. This refers to the increased excitability or responsiveness of dorsal horn neurons to an afferent input. An alteration between vertebral segments may produce a biomechanical overload leading to the alteration of signalling from mechanically or chemically sensitive neurons in paraspinal tissues. These changes in afferent input are believed to alter neural integration either by directly affecting reflex activity and/or by affecting central neural integration within motor and neuronal pools (Pickar, 2002).

Denslow, Korr and Krems (1947) were one of the first groups to investigate this phenomenon, and their findings suggested that motor neurons could be held in a facilitated state because of sensory bombardment from segmentally related dysfunctional musculature. It has been shown that central facilitation increases the receptive field of central neurons and allows innocuous mechanical stimuli access to central pain pathways (Woolf, 1994). Essentially, this means that sub-threshold stimuli may become painful as a result of increased central sensitisation. Spinal manipulation is believed to be able to overcome this facilitation by making biomechanical changes to the joint (Pickar, 2002) and/or by creating a barrage of afferent inputs into the spinal cord from muscle spindle and small-diameter afferents, ultimately silencing motor neurons (Korr, 1975).

Melzack and Wall's (1965) Gate Control Theory describes the dorsal horn of the spinal cord as having a gate-like mechanism which not only relays sensory messages but also modulates them. Nociceptive afferents from small-diameter Aγ and C fibres tend to open this gate, and non-nociceptive large diameter Aβ fibres (from joint capsule mechanoreceptor, secondary muscle spindle afferents and cutaneous mechanoreceptors) tend to close the gate to the central transmission of pain. This modulation takes place in the lamina of the dorsal horn. Simplistically, Aβ afferents enter lamina II and V, stimulating an inhibitory interneuron in lamina II (which connects to lamina V); Aγ and C fibres enter lamina V. Consequently, the central transmission of pain is a balance between the influences of these opposing stimuli (Potter, McCarthy and Oldham, 2005; Kandel, Schwartz and Jessell, 2000). HVLAT may modulate the pain gate mechanism in the dorsal horn by producing a barrage of non-nociceptive input from large diameter myelinated Aβ afferents from muscle spindles and facet joint mechanoreceptors to inhibit nociceptive C fibres (Besson and Chaouch, 1987).

## Cortical/Motoneuronal Effects

Dishman, Ball and Burke (2002) published an article which questioned some of their own previous research findings. In this subsequent paper, the authors stated that the H-reflex technique is susceptible to the effects of pre-synaptic inhibition of the afferent arm of the reflex pathway. So, by using transcranial magnetic stimulation to directly measure the effect of corticospinal inputs on the alpha motor neuron pool, they were able to perform an experiment which showed a transient (20–60 s) increase in alpha motor neuron excitability post manipulation. This paper lends further support to the theory that spinal manipulation produces a brief activation of the alpha motor neuron leading to brief muscle contraction.

Descending pathways also influence pain perception. Stimulation of the periaqueductal grey produces analgesia via the descending PAG pathways (Morgan, 1991). Stimulation of the dorsal PAG (dPAG) in the brain produces selective analgesia to mechano-nociception, whereas temperature nociception is modulated via the ventral PAG (vPAG). It is also known that sympathoexcitation results from stimulation of the dPAG, in contrast to sympatho-inhibition which occurs as a result of stimulating vPAG (Morgan, 1991). Activation of the descending dPAG is a possible mechanism for the antinociceptive effects of spinal manipulation. Sterling, Jull and Wright (2001) measured changes in pain and sympathetic outflow by comparing a C5/6 HVLA to a sham intervention (manual contact but with no movement). The authors demonstrated that HVLA produced mechanical hypoalgesia, measured by an increase in pain pressure threshold, and increased sympathetic outflow, measured by decreased blood flow, decreased skin temperature and increased skin conductance. However, there was no alteration to thermal pain thresholds. Given such selective mechanical antinociception and sympathoexcitation, this supports the theory that the mechanism of effect is due to activation of the dPAG descending pain mechanism. Vincenzino, Collins and Wright (1998) conducted a similar experiment on subjects with epicondylitis and showed again that cervical spine HVLA led to selective analgesia to mechanical stimulus and sympathoexcitation, adding further weight to the argument that spinal manipulation may influence the perception of pain by activation of the descending dPAG. This does not prove conclusively that there is definitely direct activation of dPAG, only that the effects of HVLA give similar findings to what would be expected with stimulation of the dPAG. Therefore, there is a plausible link between the two, and it is inferred that HVLA may lead to stimulation of the dPAG.

## References

Besson, J.-M. and Chaouch, A. (1987). Peripheral and spinal mechanisms of nociception. *Physiology Review, 67*(1), 67–186.

Denslow, J.S., Korr, I.M. and Krems, A.D. (1947). Quantitative studies of chronic facilitation in human motoneuron pools. *American Journal of Physiology, 150*, 229–38.

Dishman, J.D., Ball, K.A. and Burke, J. (2002). Central motor excitability changes after spinal manipulation: A transcranial magnetic stimulation study. *Journal of Manipulative and Physiological Therapeutics, 25*, 1–10.

Kandel, E.R., Schwartz, J.H. and Jessell, T.M. (2000). *Principles of Neural Science*, 4th edition. London: McGraw-Hill.

Korr, I.M. (1975). Proprioceptors and somatic dysfunction. *Journal of the American Osteopathic Association, 74*, 638–650.

Melzack, R. and Wall, P.D. (1965). Pain mechanisms: A new theory. *Science, 150*, 971–979.

Morgan, M.M. (1991). Differences in antinociception evoked from dorsal and ventral regions of the caudal periaqueductal gray matter. In A. Depaulis and R. Bandlier (Eds), *The Midbrain Periaqueductal Gray Matter*. New York, NY: Plenum.

Pickar, J.G. (2002). Neurophysiological effects of spinal manipulation. *The Spine Journal* 2, 357–371.

Potter, L., McCarthy, C. and Oldham, J. (2005). Physiological effects of spinal manipulation: A review of proposed theories. *Physical Therapy Reviews, 10*, 163–170.

Sterling, M., Jull, G. and Wright, A. (2001). Cervical mobilisation: Concurrent effects on pain, sympathetic nervous system activity and motor activity. *Manual Therapy 6*, 72–81.

Vincenzino, B., Collins, D. and Wright, A. (1998). An investigation of the interrelationship between manipulative therapy-induced hypoalgesia and sympathoexcitation. *Journal of Manipulative and Physiological Therapeutics, 21*, 448–453.

Woolf, C.J. (1994). The dorsal horn: State-dependent sensory processing and the generation of pain. In P.D. Wall and R. Melzack (Eds), *Textbook of Pain*, 3rd edition. Edinburgh: Churchill Livingstone.

# CHAPTER 3

# The Effects of Manipulation on Fascia

## Introduction

Fascia is an uninterrupted network throughout the body which has the ability to adjust its elasticity and consistency under tension (Findley *et al.*, 2012). There are various forms of manual therapies that have been developed to work on the fascia for therapeutic purposes. Although these therapies have considerable variation in their techniques, they can be broadly divided into two major groups: myofascial release (e.g. soft-tissue manipulation) and manipulative techniques (e.g. high-velocity, low-amplitude thrust) (Simmonds, Miller and Gemmell, 2012). In general, these techniques are used to treat a variety of musculoskeletal as well as visceral problems, including sprains, tendonitis, peripheral neuropathy, neck pain syndromes, gastritis, abdominal pain, constipation, menstrual cramps and irritable bowel syndrome (Stecco and Stecco, 2010).

Scientific research on these techniques continues; so far, a number of positive clinical findings have been reported (Pedrelli, Stecco and Day, 2009; Day, Stecco and Stecco, 2009; Oulianova, 2011; Harper, Steinbeck and Aron, 2016). However, although the volume of research on these techniques has increased significantly in recent years, little is yet understood about their effects on fascia. Even though many authors have claimed to change the density, tonus, viscosity or arrangement of fascia through the application of manual techniques (Cantu and Grodin, 1992;

Ward, 1993; Paoletti, 2002), their proposed explanations predominantly allude to the fascia's ability to adapt to physical stress.

Given the lack of firm theories based on scientific evidence, this chapter is written to review the current theories of the effects of manipulative therapies on fascia. In addition, current understandings about the apparently confounding fascia and its role in human body are also discussed.

**What is Fascia?**

Fascia is the largest component of white fibrous tissue that extends over the whole body just below the skin. It is a continuous sheet – composed of connective tissue – enveloping and yet at the same time compartmentalising all parts of the body (O'Connell, 2003). It forms an extensive, membranous continuum, a 3D whole-body matrix of structural support, and is an interconnected network of fibrous collagenous tissues, which moves, connects and senses all of the body's vital organs, nerve fibres, blood vessels, muscles and bones (Thomas and Robet, 2009).

Fascia provides ongoing physiological support for the body's metabolically active systems composed of specialised cells and tissues (McGechie, 2010). It has the function of connecting, communicating and coordinating all parts of the body in its entirety (Langevin, 2006). The structural integrity of fascia is also essential, as it assists in response to mechanical stress and the maintenance of posture and locomotion (O'Connell, 2003; Stecco and Stecco, 2010). In summary, the fascia supports the body in a number of ways, such as by increasing joint stability, facilitating movement, assisting in the repair of tissue damage, protecting against infection and contributing to haemodynamic and biochemical processes (LeMoon, 2008).

Fascia has three layers: superficial, deep (muscle) and subserous (visceral).

**Table 3.1 Different layers of fascia**

| Name | Characteristics |
|---|---|
| Superficial fascia | • a web of collagen with a membranous appearance<br>• forms a protective covering all over the body<br>• composed of the subcutaneous connective tissue containing elastin, collagen as well as some fat tissue<br>• absent in the face, palms of the hand and soles of the feet |
| Deep fascia | • a layer of fibrous connective tissue that sheaths all muscles<br>• devoid of fat tissues and forms compartments for cavities, organs and structures<br>• envelops all bones, including various organs and glands, and becomes specialised in muscles and nerves |
| Visceral fascia | • a thin, fibrous membrane composed mostly of reticular fibres<br>• covers, supports and lubricates organs<br>• wraps muscle in layers of connective tissue membranes |

Sources: O'Connell (2003); Lancerotto *et al.* (2011); Findley *et al.* (2012)

# Effects of Manipulative Therapies on Fascia

### Mechanical Effects

Manipulative therapies have long been hypothesised to produce mechanical effects on fascia (Paoletti, 2002; Ward, 1993; Cantu and Grodin, 1992). These therapies are thought to improve balance, motion and posture by changing the mechanical properties of the fascia, such as density, tonus, arrangement and viscosity (Smith, 2005; Stanborough, 2004; DellaGrotte *et al.*, 2008). However, most of these theories are mainly based on the fascia's ability to adapt to physical stresses, and its role in transmitting mechanical forces between muscles (Huijing, 2009).

Fascia tightens and loses its flexibility due to acute inflammation; it may also shorten because of long-term postural positioning, which hinders its full excursion. When fascial tightness or shortness occurs, stretching of fascia might result pain at distant sensitive areas of the body – for example, blood vessels and nerves (Findley *et al.*, 2012). Osteopathic physicians and manual therapists claim that once fascial tightness is released through appropriate application of a manipulative technique, pressure is eased from these sensitive areas and blood circulation returns to normal range (Walton, 2008; Findley *et al.*, 2012). Some manual therapists have also reported palpable tissue release after applying a soft-tissue manipulation to dense fascial areas (Juhan, 1987; Ward, 1993; Stecco, 2004). These palpable sensations of tissue release have been attributed as a breaching of fascial cross-links, a transition from viscous gel state to less viscous sol state in the extracellular matrix, and other passive viscoelastic changes of fasciae (Stanborough, 2004; Juhan, 1987; Stecco, 2004).

However, this explanation of palpable viscoelastic changes in human fasciae has been highly controversial, because it is not yet known whether the applied mechanical force and duration of a given manipulative technique can be sufficient to cause such an effect. Although some authors (Sucher *et al.*, 2005; Stecco, 2004) have supported the explanation, others (Threlkeld, 1992; Schleip, 2003b) have argued against it. Chaudhry *et al.* (2008) have done a comprehensive study on this question. They found that fascia lata and plantar fascia are very stiff and require very large forces to produce even 1% compression and 1% shear. In contrast, they showed that under strong forces, deformation of softer tissues, such as superficial nasal fascia, is possible. Taken together, Chaudhry *et al.* dismissed the idea that palpable tissue release might result from deformation in the firm tissues of plantar fascia and fascia lata. Instead, they proposed that these palpable effects are more likely the result of reflexive alterations, such as tonus changes, in the softer tissue or changes in twisting or extension forces in the tissue.

In summary, it can be said that more research is needed to fully explore the mechanical effects of manipulation on fascia.

## Piezoelectric Effects

The charge-based mechanism has long been used to explain the effects of manipulative therapy on fascia. This theory considers that fascia has piezoelectric properties; hence, it can transduce mechanical force into electric energy and serve as a communication medium between the inner and outer environment (Barnes, 1997; Simmonds *et al.*, 2012). The theory postulates that fascia's piezoelectric effects predominantly cause the alterations in its mechanical properties before and after manipulative therapies (Findley *et al.*, 2012).

O'Connell (2003) provided a bioelectric model to explain this theory. According to the author, when compressive and distraction forces result in trauma in the musculoskeletal system, a chain of events is triggered by bioelectric potential changes in the collagen-laden fascia. These bioelectric changes also affect the extracellular fluid (ECF) components. Consequently, the ECF components alter in charge and polarity, and eventually affect the motion of the fascia. O'Connell suggested that this somatic dysfunction, whether initiated by internal or external trauma, could be normalised by the manual application of osteopathic manipulative techniques, particularly by the myofascial release techniques. These techniques involve applying compressive and distraction forces into the stressed tissues. To identify altered patterns of fascial motion, these forces are aimed near or distant from a restricted to normal motion. When the restriction or point of ease is met by the technique, the fascia responds rapidly via its collagen fibres by creating microelectric potential changes. As a result, the fascial restrictions decrease and motion resumes.

In contrast to this theory, there has been argument for years about whether fascia is actually a piezoelectric material or not (Ahn and Grodzinsky, 2009; Findley, 2011). However, Rivard *et al.* (2011) recently used second harmonic generation (SHG) microscopy to demonstrate that fascia has noncentrosymmetric (piezoelectric) structures. The authors also described fascia as a nanometric randomly poled crystal. On the other hand, Langevin (2006), though not dismissing the piezoelectric effects of fascia, noted that the evidence is still very limited. In addition, the author argued that it is not yet known whether fascia actually transmits microelectric potentials in vivo and, even if it does, whether these bioelectric changes are significant to make biomechanical changes.

Taken together, in light of the above discussion, it can be said that even though the piezoelectric theory of fascia is not yet proven, fascial piezoelectricity can be a fruitful area of research. Therefore, more studies in this field are required to determine whether the piezoelectric effects of fascia have significant clinical relevance.

## Neurophysiological Effects

The neurophysiological mechanism is a widely discussed concept among researchers to explain both the immediate and sustained fascial responsiveness to manipulative therapies. The concept received the attention of the broader scientific community when Cottingham (1985) proposed that sensory Golgi receptors within the fascial fibres could be stimulated by soft-tissue manipulation. The author suggested that during slow stretching of the myofascial tissues, these receptors respond by reducing the firing rate of specific alpha motor neurons, which ultimately leads to tonus changes of the related tissues. Although some authors (Schleip, 1989; Ward, 1993) readily appreciated the concept, later studies have shown that such stimulation of Golgi receptors is not possible via passive stretching (Jami, 1992; Lederman, 1997). Lederman (1997) suggested that this activation could occur only when the muscle fibres are in active contractions. However, Schleip (2003a) did not discard the possibility of Golgi receptor stimulation by stronger deep tissue manipulation. The author speculated that deep tissue work could indeed influence these receptors, as 90% of them are less explored – and located outside the Golgi tendon.

Another pioneering model that has been highly cited to explain the neurophysiological mechanism is fascial plasticity, which is proposed by Schleip (2003a, 2003b). This model is based on the early work of Yahia *et al.* (1992), which showed that fascia is densely populated by mechanoreceptors that consist of three groups. Schleip (2003a) presumed that the Pacini corpuscles of the first group might be influenced by high-velocity low-amplitude (HVLA) manipulation, whereas Ruffini corpuscles of the second group respond to slow myofascial techniques, which involve tangential forces – that is, lateral stretch. The third group of mechanoreceptors are interstitial receptors (type III and IV afferents), which have been shown to possess autonomic functions. Schleip (2003a) proposed that soft-tissue manipulation stimulates intrafascial mechanoreceptors to influence the proprioception. The author hypothesised that stimulation of these mechanoreceptors results in transmission of altered proprioceptive signals to the central nervous system (CNS). When these inputs are transmitted to the brain, the CNS then responds by resetting the gamma motor system, which ultimately leads to changes in muscle tonus regulation. Furthermore, Schleip (2003b) suggested that stimulation of mechanoreceptors, such as Ruffini endings and interstitial receptors, could trigger changes in sympathetic tone and/or local vasodilation.

The fascial plasticity model by Schleip was intended for soft-tissue therapies. However, after reviewing Schleip's work, Simmonds *et al.* (2012) proposed that this model might be readily adopted for HVLA manipulation as well. Simmonds *et al.* hypothesised that the basis for the neurophysiological mechanisms of soft-tissue and HVLA manipulation are the same, and considered that these two therapies are at two ends of a continuous spectrum of effects. In addition, referring to the autonomic involvement of the spinal manipulative therapies, they suggested that Schleip's proposed separate 'loops' in the feedback pathway of the CNS and autonomic nervous system (ANS) are linked by the dorsal periaqueductal grey (dPAG).

Although the exact details of fascial neurodynamics have not yet been fully explored, in light of the above discussion, it can be said that fascia may have a key role in nociception and mechanoreception. However, more research is needed to establish the neurophysiological mechanism of fascia.

## Conclusion

This chapter reviews three possible effects of manual therapies on fascia. Even though none of the effects discussed here is yet established, based on our review we can confirm that the ability of manual therapies to affect fascia has some support from the current literature. However, more studies in this field are required to determine the efficacy and effects of manual therapies on fascia.

## References

Ahn, A.C. and Grodzinsky, A.J. (2009). Relevance of collagen piezoelectricity to 'Wolff's Law': A critical review. *Medical Engineering and Physics, 31*(7), 733–741.

Barnes, M.F. (1997). The basic science of myofascial release: Morphologic change in connective tissue. *Journal of Bodywork and Movement Therapies, 1*(4), 231–238.

Cantu, R.I. and Grodin, A.J. (1992). *Myofascial Manipulation: Theory and Clinical Application.* Gaithersburg, MD: Aspen Publishers.

Chaudhry, H., Schleip, R., Ji, Z., Bukict, B., Maney, M. and Findley, T. (2008). Three-dimensional mathematical model for deformation of human fasciae in manual therapy. *The Journal of the American Osteopathic Association, 108*(8), 379–390.

Cottingham, J.T. (1985). *Healing through Touch: A History and a Review of the Physiological Evidence.* Rolf Institute.

Day, J.A., Stecco, C. and Stecco, A. (2009). Application of Fascial Manipulation© technique in chronic shoulder pain – Anatomical basis and clinical implications. *Journal of Bodywork and Movement Therapies, 13*(2), 128–135.

DellaGrotte, J., Ridi, R., Landi, M. and Stephens, J. (2008). Postural improvement using core integration to lengthen myofascia. *Journal of Bodywork and Movement Therapies, 12*(3), 231–245.

Findley, T., Chaudhry, H., Stecco, A. and Roman, M. (2012). Fascia research: A narrative review. *Journal of Bodywork and Movement Therapies, 16*(1), 67–75.

Findley, T.W, (2011). Fascia research from a clinician/scientist's perspective. *International Journal of Therapeutic Massage and Bodywork, 4*(4), 1.

Harper, B., Steinbeck, L. and Aron, A. (2016). The effect of adding Fascial Manipulation® to the physical therapy plan of care for low back pain patients. *Journal of Bodywork and Movement Therapies, 1*(20), 148–149.

Huijing, P.A. (2009). Epimuscular myofascial force transmission: A historical review and implications for new research. International Society of Biomechanics Muybridge Award Lecture, Taipei, 2007. *Journal of Biomechanics, 42*(1), 9–21.

Jami, L. (1992). Golgi tendon organs in mammalian skeletal muscle: Functional properties and central actions. *Physiological Reviews, 72*(3), 623–666.

Juhan, D. (1987). *Job's Body: A Handbook for Bodywork.* Barrytown, NY: Station Hill Press.

Lancerotto, L., Stecco, C., Macchi, V., Porzionato, A., Stecco, A. and De Caro, R. (2011). Layers of the abdominal wall: Anatomical investigation of subcutaneous tissue and superficial fascia. *Surgical and Radiologic Anatomy, 33*(10), 835–842.

Langevin, H.M. (2006). Connective tissue: A body-wide signaling network. *Medical Hypotheses, 66*(6), 1074–1077.

Lederman, E. (1997). *Fundamentals of Manual Therapy.* Edinburgh: Churchill Livingstone.

LeMoon, K. (2008). Terminology used in fascia research. *Journal of Bodywork and Movement Therapies, 12*(3), 204–212.

McGechie, D. (2010). The connective tissue hypothesis for acupuncture mechanisms. *Journal of Chinese Medicine, 93*, 14.

O'Connell, J.A. (2003). Bioelectric responsiveness of fascia: A model for understanding the effects of manipulation. *Techniques in Orthopaedics, 18*(1), 67–73.

Oulianova, I. (2011). *An Investigation into the Effects of Fascial Manipulation on Dysmenorrhea* (Doctoral dissertation, RMTBC).

Paoletti, S. (2002). *Les fascias: Role des tissues dans la mecanique humaine.* Sully.

Pedrelli, A., Stecco, C. and Day, J.A. (2009). Treating patellar tendinopathy with Fascial Manipulation. *Journal of Bodywork and Movement Therapies, 13*(1), 73–80.

Rivard, M., Laliberté, M., Bertrand-Grenier, A., Harnagea, C., Pfeffer, C.P., Vallières, M., St-Pierre, Y., Pignolet, A., El Khakani, M.A. and Légaré, F. (2011). The structural origin of second harmonic generation in fascia. *Biomedical Optics Express, 2*(1), 26–36.

Schleip, R. (1989). A new explanation of the effect of Rolfing. *Rolf Lines, 15*(1), 18–20.

Schleip, R. (2003a). Fascial plasticity: A new neurobiological explanation: Part 1. *Journal of Bodywork and Movement Therapies, 7*(1), 11–19.

Schleip, R. (2003b). Fascial plasticity: A new neurobiological explanation Part 2. *Journal of Bodywork and Movement Therapies, 7*(2), 104–116.

Simmonds, N., Miller, P. and Gemmell, H. (2012). A theoretical framework for the role of fascia in manual therapy. *Journal of Bodywork and Movement Therapies, 16*(1), 83–93.

Smith, J. (2005). *Structural Bodywork*. Edinburgh: Elselvier.

Stanborough, M. (2004). *Direct Release Myofascial Technique: An Illustrated Guide for Practitioners*. Churchill Livingstone.

Stecco, L. and Stecco, A. (2010). *The Fascial Manipulation© Technique and its biomechanical model – a guide to the human fascial system*. Available at http://citeseerx.ist.psu.edu/viewdoc/download?doi=10.1.1.608.5164&rep=rep1&type=pdf (accessed 27 March 2016).

Stecco, L. (2004). *Fascial Manipulation for Musculoskeletal Pain*. Padova: Piccin.

Sucher, B.M., Hinrichs, R.N., Welcher, R.L., Quiroz, L.D., Laurent, B.F.S. and Morrison, B.J. (2005). Manipulative treatment of carpal tunnel syndrome: Biomechanical and osteopathic intervention to increase the length of the transverse carpal ligament: Part 2. Effect of sex differences and manipulative 'priming'. *The Journal of the American Osteopathic Association, 105*(3), 135–143.

Thomas, F. and Robet, S. (2009). *Introduction in Fascia Research II, Amsterdam Basic Science and Implications for Conventional and Complementary Health Care*. Elsevier Press.

Threlkeld, A.J. (1992). The effects of manual therapy on connective tissue. *Physical Therapy, 72*(12), 893–902.

Walton, A. (2008). Efficacy of myofascial release techniques in the treatment of primary Raynaud's phenomenon. *Journal of Bodywork and Movement Therapies, 12*(3), 274–280.

Ward, R.C. (1993). Myofascial release concepts. In V. Basmajian and R. Nyberg (Eds), *Rational Manual Therapies*. Baltimore, MD: Williams & Wilkins.

Yahia, L.H., Rhalmi, S., Newman, N. and Isler, M. (1992). Sensory innervation of human thoracolumbar fascia: An immunohistochemical study. *Acta Orthopaedica Scandinavica, 63*(2), 195–197.

# CHAPTER 4

# Safety and Patient Screening

## Introduction

Manipulation is an alternative form of intervention to treat musculoskeletal conditions. It is considered relatively safe and effective when administered skilfully and appropriately. However, as with all interventions, there are known risks and contraindications to manipulation as well. Although the frequency of severe adverse events is very low (Coulter, 1998), certain conditions require special caution to be exercised while performing manipulative procedures. These include, for example, vascular disease, osteoporosis, disc herniation, nerve injury and vertebral artery syndrome (Ernst, 2007).

Over the past decades, protocols or clinical guidelines have been developed to assist the practitioner in identifying patients at risk (Rivett, Thomas and Bolton, 2005). The protocols include absolute contraindications and red flag symptoms in which manipulation should never be performed. In addition, there are relative contraindications where the intervention or procedure is modified so that the recipient is not at an unwarranted risk (Puentedura et al., 2012).

Prevention of complications can be further facilitated if sound clinical judgement is practised, adequate skill is exercised and quality care is provided. It is also of significant importance that when onset of a complication is associated with a manipulative procedure, the intervention should not be repeated (Refshauge et al., 2002).

Elements for determining the appropriateness of a manipulation technique include detailed history-taking, thorough physical examination and adequate evaluation of the recipient's pre-existing and presenting condition (Rivett *et al.*, 2005). Several provocative testing procedures are performed to determine the safety and efficacy of a manipulation technique. These include laboratory tests, skeletal imaging, orthopaedic and neurological examinations, as well as observational and tactile assessments. Good clinical management involves timely re-evaluation of the patient's progress during the course of the treatment, effective practitioner–patient communication, supportive and adjunctive measures, rehabilitative and preventive exercises, and patient education and counselling (World Health Organization, 2005).

The existing risk assessment protocols and guidelines, however, have been subjected to critical reviews in recent years (Rivett *et al.*, 2005). The adequacy of the pre-manipulative provocative tests is questioned (Refshauge, 2001), because a number of studies have demonstrated a high rate of both false positive and false negative results (Bolton, Stick and Lord, 1989; Cote *et al.*, 1995; Westaway, Stratford and Symons, 2003). It has been identified that this inconsistency in test results is largely due to the lack of accurate and reliable screening tools (Puentedura *et al.*, 2012). As a result, the goal to establish adequate guidelines for standards of practice and develop acceptable preventive strategies is yet not achieved.

The aim of this chapter is to review complications of and contraindications to manipulation that have been suggested so far and illustrate various clinical conditions that require treatment modification.

## Complications of Spinal Manipulation

Spinal manipulation has been a safe and effective means of treating a variety of biomechanical problems of the spine. As with all conventional treatments, manipulation also has the potential to cause complications, but the risk of serious adverse events following a manipulative procedure is so far unknown (Di Fabio, 1999).

## Causes of Complications and Adverse Events

- Lack of knowledge
- Misdiagnosis
- Insufficient examination
- Poor clinical judgement
- Poor interprofessional cooperation
- Inappropriate technique application
- Lack of rational attitude and technique
- Unnecessary or excessive use of manipulation
- Cervical manipulation
- Presence of a herniated nucleus pulposus
- Presence of arteriosclerotic disease
- Presence of coagulation dyscrasias

Sources: Shekelle *et al.* (1991); Henderson (1992); Refshauge *et al.* (2002)

Chiropractors tend to downplay the risks of life-threatening complications due to manipulation (Killinger, 2004) and often attribute those to poor clinical judgement, inadequate skill or inappropriate use of techniques (Haneline and Triano, 2005). However, several recent systematic reviews have highlighted a range of serious adverse events following cervical spine manipulation and suggest that serious complications do exist (Ernst, 2007; Gouveia, Castanho and Ferreira, 2009; Puentedura *et al.*, 2012). Nevertheless, many of these concerns have been derived from epidemiologic inference, and the reports of serious complications have primarily been based on case reports and prospective or retrospective studies. Furthermore, based on the estimates done in the published literature, it has repeatedly been suggested that the frequency of these incidences is rare (Coulter, 1998; Haldeman *et al.*, 2001; Gouveia *et al.*, 2009). As a result, the cause-and-effect relationship between manipulation and such adverse events is yet not established.

## Table 4.1 Adverse consequences of spinal manipulation

| Severity | Complications | Frequency | Reference |
|---|---|---|---|
| Mild to moderate | <ul><li>Localised discomfort</li><li>Weakness</li><li>Increased pain</li><li>Radiation of pain</li><li>Paraesthesia</li><li>Headaches</li><li>Visual disturbance</li><li>Stiffness</li><li>Fatigue</li><li>Vertigo</li><li>Loss of consciousness</li></ul> | About 33–61% | Gouveia *et al.* (2009) |
| Serious | <ul><li>Stroke</li><li>Vertebral artery dissection</li><li>Internal carotid artery dissection</li><li>Myelopathy</li><li>Pathological fractures</li><li>Dural tear</li><li>Costochondral separation</li><li>Rib fracture</li><li>Disc herniation</li><li>Cauda equina syndrome</li><li>Vascular accident</li><li>Death</li></ul> | Extremely rare | Ernst (2007); World Health Organization (2005) |

In general, complications following a spinal manipulation range from non-serious side effects, such as localised discomfort, fatigue or headache, to serious adverse events, such as stroke, vascular accidents or death (Refshauge *et al.*, 2002). Minor side effects from a manipulative procedure are relatively common and may occur in up to 55% of patients (Senstad, Leboeuf-Yde and Borchgrevink, 1997). However, most of these adverse issues are self-limiting and often resolve within 24–48 hours (Cagnie *et al.*, 2004). Conversely, serious complications of manipulation are considered to be extremely rare (Triano, 2001). The precise incidence of such adverse events is yet not known, but estimates of risks have been reported to vary widely between studies (see Tables 4.2 and 4.3).

The most serious adverse event frequently reported in these studies is vertebral artery dissection, which has been thought to result from over-stretching of the artery during rotational manipulation (Nadgir *et al.*, 2003). Ernst (2007) suggests that this seems to occur at the level of the atlantoaxial joint and involve the vertebrobasilar system, particularly the distal loop of the vertebral artery. The incidence of vertebral artery dissection, however, is considered to be rare. The calculated rate of incidence is 1 per 5.85 million cervical manipulations (Haldeman *et al.*, 2002).

**Table 4.2 Rate of serious adverse events due to spinal manipulation**

| Rate of complications | Manipulated region of the spine | Authors |
| --- | --- | --- |
| 1 per 1.3 million | Cervical spine | Klougart, Leboeuf-Yde and Rasmussen (1996) |
| 1 per 8.06 million | Cervical spine | Haldeman *et al.* (2001) |
| 1 per 50,000 | Cervical spine | Magarey *et al.* (2004) |
| 1.46 per 10 million | Not mentioned (represented the whole spine) | Gouveia *et al.* (2009) |
| 6.39 per 10 million | Cervical spine | Coulter (1998) |
| 1 per 100 million | Lumbar spine | Coulter (1998) |

**Table 4.3 Nature of serious complications following spinal manipulation**

| Nature of complication | Frequency of incidence | Reference |
| --- | --- | --- |
| Vertebral artery dissection | 1 per 5.85 million cervical manipulations | Haldeman *et al.* (2002) |
| Cerebrovascular accident | 1 per 0.9 million upper cervical spine manipulation | Klougart *et al.* (1996) |
| Cerebrovascular accident | 1 per 100,000 chiropractic office visits | Rothwell, Bondy and Williams (2001) |
| Neurovascular compromise | 1 per 50,000 to 1 per 5 million manipulations | Rivett and Milburn (1996) |
| Stroke | 5 per 100,000 manipulations | Gouveia *et al.* (2009) |
| Stroke | 1 per 163,000 cervical spine manipulations | Rivett and Reid (1998) |
| Stroke | 1 per 200,000 cervical spine manipulations | Haynes (1994) |
| Death | 2.68 per 10 million manipulations | Coulter *et al.* (1996); Gouveia *ct al.* (2009) |

To put things in perspective, some authors have compared the frequency of serious incidences for manipulation with other forms of conventional therapy for the same conditions. In comparison, Coulter (1998) suggests that the use of spinal manipulation is far safer than conservative treatments: non-steroidal anti-inflammatory drugs (NSAIDs) are associated with 3.2 complications per 1000 patients and cervical spine surgery has 15.6 cases of complication per 1000 surgeries. Furthermore, Dabbs and Lauretti (1995) stated that the incidence of serious adverse event or death associated with NSAID use is 100–400 times higher than that of the spinal manipulation.

In contrast, Ernst (2007) argued that the incidence figures might be over-optimistic or nonsensical, because none of these reports considered under-reporting of incidences, while under-reporting was found to be close to 100% (Dupeyron *et al.*, 2003; Stevinson *et al.*, 2001). The author also suggested that if under-reporting was taken into consideration, this might significantly distort the incidence figures.

Taken together, in light of the above evidence, it can be said that spinal manipulation is certainly associated with serious complications but the risk of serious adverse events is statistically low. However, even though serious complications of manipulation might well be minor, in matters of patients' safety the risk of vascular accidents, stroke or death is not negligible. To admit best interests of the recipient, the practitioners should therefore perform a thorough and meticulous pre-manipulative examination to rule out all contraindications and red flag symptoms so that the patient is not at unwarranted risk.

## Contraindications to Spinal Manipulation

There are a number of contraindications to spinal manipulation. These range from an inappropriate condition for such an intervention, where the patient is not likely to benefit from the procedure, to a risky condition, where manipulation may result in life-threatening complications. These contraindications are provided to help practitioners with decision-making so that they do not place a patient at risk of a serious complication following spinal manipulation.

**Note:** The presence of a contraindicated condition in one area of the spine does not mean that spinal manipulation should not be used in other areas. In many instances, manipulation is contraindicated in one area of the spine, yet it has shown to be favourable for another region (Gatterman, 1992).

### Absolute and Relative Contraindications
In general, clinical contraindications to manipulation can be divided into absolute, where manipulation should not be performed because it can place a patient at risk for an adverse event, and relative, where the intervention should be modified and provided with appropriate

care so that the patient is not at undue risk. Absolute contraindications comprise a number of diseases and conditions, including bone diseases, congenital conditions, metabolic processes, vertebrobasilar arterial insufficiency, spinal cord compression, and many more (see Table 4.4). Relative contraindications include inflammatory joint processes, minor osteoporosis, disc prolapse and protrusion, hypermobility or ligamentous laxity, spondylolisthesis, degenerative joint diseases, to name a few (see Table 4.5).

## Table 4.4 Absolute contraindications for spinal manipulation

| Authors | Contraindicated diseases or conditions |
|---|---|
| World Health Organization (2005); Gibbons and Tehan (2004); Liem and Dobler (2014); Wainapel and Fast (2003); Koss (1990) | **Articular derangement**<br>• Inflammatory conditions (e.g. rheumatoid arthritis, seronegative spondyloarthropathies such as ankylosing spondylitis, reactive arthritis or psoriatic arthritis, demineralisation or ligamentous laxity with anatomical subluxation or dislocation)<br>• Fractures and dislocations, or healed fractures with signs of ligamentous rupture or instability<br>• Atlantoaxial instability<br><br>**Note:** Subacute and chronic ankylosing spondylitis and other chronic arthropathies without any signs of ligamentous laxity, anatomic subluxation or ankylosis are not contraindicated at the area of pathology.<br><br>**Bone diseases**<br>• Active juvenile avascular necrosis (particularly of the joints that bear weight of the body)<br>• *Acute infections* (e.g. osteomyelitis, bone tuberculosis and septic discitis)<br>• Metabolic (osteomalacia)<br>• Anomalies (e.g. spina bifida, dens hypoplasia, dysplasia, diastematomyelia, deformations of the spine, unstable os odontoideum)<br>• Tumour-like and dysphasic bone lesions<br>• Iatrogenic (*long treatment with cortisone*)<br><br>**Tumours, metastases**<br>• Spinal cord tumour<br>• Malignant bone tumour<br>• Meningeal tumour<br>• *Aggressive types of benign tumours (e.g. an aneurismal bone cyst, giant cell tumour, osteoblastoma or osteoid osteoma)* |

**Neurological disorders**

- *Frank disc herniation with accompanying signs of neurological deficit*
- Cervical myelopathy
- Meningitis
- Spinal cord compression
- Nerve compression syndrome
- Intracranial hypertension
- Cauda equina syndrome
- Hydrocephalus of unknown aetiology

**Vascular disorders**

- *Serious bleeding diathesis (haemophilia, anticoagulation)*
- Insufficiency/stenosis of the vertebral/carotid artery
- *Vertebrobasilar insufficiency syndrome*
- *Vascular calcification of the arterial walls*
- Arterial tortuosity syndrome
- *Aortic aneurysm*

## Table 4.5 Relative contraindications

| Mentioned by some authors | Contraindicated diseases or conditions |
|---|---|
| Croibier and Meddeb (2006); Cagnie *et al.* (2004); Thanvi *et al.* (2005) | **Vascular and morphological pathology** <br>• Venous thrombosis <br>• Angina pectoris <br>• Signs of arteriosclerotic disease, either direct or indirect <br>• High levels of homocysteine <br>• *Past history of heart attack* <br>• Abnormalities of the lumbosacral/craniocervical junction (e.g. basilar invagination) <br>• Vertebral osteosynthesis |
| Greenman (2005) | • Genetic disorders (e.g. *Down syndrome*) |
| World Health Organization (2005) | • Haematomas, whether intracanalicular or spinal cord <br>• Dislocation of a vertebra <br>• Neoplastic disease of muscle or other soft tissue <br>• Positive Kernig's or Lhermitte's signs <br>• Arnold-Chiari malformation of the cervical spine <br>• Syringomyelia |
| Vickers and Zollman (1990) | • Acute post-traumatic instability (e.g. ligamentous rupture) |

| Mentioned by some authors | Contraindicated diseases or conditions |
|---|---|
| Giles and Singer (1997); Giles and Singer (2000) | • Congenital, generalised hypermobility<br>• Synovial cysts in the area of the thoracic spine<br>• Visceral referred pain<br>• Obvious spinal deformity<br>• General hypermobility<br>• Long-term anticoagulant therapy |
| Koss (1990) | • Acute whiplash<br>• Acute vertigo |
| Wainapel and Fast (2003) | • *Osteoporosis*<br>• *Spondylolisthesis* |

**Note:** Conditions in italics represent relative-to-absolute contraindication to manipulation at the area of pathology.

## Red Flags

Red flag symptoms for spinal manipulation (see box below) have been identified to help clinicians in making sound clinical judgements as part of the examination process. In general, these symptoms indicate the presence of a more serious underlying condition that may place the recipient at undue risk (Refshauge *et al.*, 2002). It has been recommended that red flags should be used in conjunction with contraindications to determine the appropriateness of the manipulative procedure and prevent adverse events that may result from manipulation (Childs *et al.*, 2005).

If any of the red flag symptoms mentioned below are present in a patient, the practitioner should prioritise sound clinical reasoning and exercise utmost caution, so that the patient is not placed at risk for an undue adverse event following manipulation.

## Red Flags for Spinal Manipulation

- Previous diagnosis of vertebrobasilar insufficiency
- Signs and symptoms of spondylitis and spondylolisthesis
- Previous history of joint or segment surgery
- Facial/intra-oral anaesthesia or paraesthesia
- History of long-term steroid therapy
- History of traumatic event suffering
- Women at post-menopause
- Patients with psychogenic complaints
- Patients with nystagmus
- Presence of osteopenia
- Presence of scoliosis
- Diplopia or other visual disturbances
- Ataxia of gait, coordination
- Dizziness/vertigo/giddiness/lightheadedness
- Blurred vision
- Nausea
- Sudden fall without loss of consciousness or drop attack
- Sensation of ringing or buzzing in the ears
- Presence of dysarthria
- Signs of difficulty swallowing or dysphagia
- Aggravation of any of the above symptoms during manipulation
- No improvement or worsening of symptoms following multiple manipulations

Sources: World Health Organization (2005); Puentedura *et al.* (2012)

# References

Bolton, P.S., Stick, P.E. and Lord, R.S. (1989). Failure of clinical tests to predict cerebral ischemia before neck manipulation. *Journal of Manipulative and Physiological Therapeutics, 12*(4), 304–307.

Cagnie, B., Vinck, E., Beernaert, A. and Cambier, D. (2004). How common are side effects of spinal manipulation and can these side effects be predicted? *Manual Therapy, 9*(3), 151–156.

Childs, J.D., Flynn, T.W., Fritz, J.M., Piva, S.R., Whitman, J.M., Wainner, R.S. and Greenman, P.E. (2005). Screening for vertebrobasilar insufficiency in patients with neck pain: Manual therapy decision-making in the presence of uncertainty. *Journal of Orthopaedic and Sports Physical Therapy, 35*(5), 300–306.

Cote, P., Kreitz, B.G., Cassidy, J.D. and Thiel, H. (1995). The validity of the extension-rotation test as a clinical screening procedure before neck manipulation: A secondary analysis. *Journal of Manipulative and Physiological Therapeutics, 19*(3), 159–164.

Coulter, I.D. (1998). Efficacy and risks of chiropractic manipulation: What does the evidence suggest? *Integrative Medicine, 1*(2), 61–66.

Coulter, I.D., Hurwitz, E.L., Adams, A.H., Meeker, W.C. *et al.* (1996). *The Appropriateness of Manipulation and Mobilization of the Cervical Spine.* Santa Monica, CA: Rand.

Croibier, A. and Meddeb, G. (2006). *Diagnostik in der Osteopathie.* Elsevier, Urban & Fischer.

Dabbs, V. and Lauretti, W.J. (1995). A risk assessment of cervical manipulation vs. NSAIDs for the treatment of neck pain. *Journal of Manipulative and Physiological Therapeutics, 18*(8), 530–536.

Di Fabio, R.P. (1999). Manipulation of the cervical spine: Risks and benefits. *Physical Therapy, 79*(1), 50–65.

Dupeyron, A., Vautravers, P., Lecocq, J. and Isner-Horobeti, M.E. (2003). [Complications following vertebral manipulation: A survey of a French region physicians]. *Annales de readaptation et de medécine physique: revue scientifique de la Societe francaise de reeducation fonctionnelle de readaptation et de medecine physique, 46*(1), 33–40.

Ernst, E. (2007). Adverse effects of spinal manipulation: A systematic review. *Journal of the Royal Society of Medicine, 100*(7), 330–338.

Gatterman, M. (1992). *Standards for Contraindications to Spinal Manipulative Therapy. Chiropractic Standards of Practice and Quality of Care.* Gaithersburg, MD: Aspen Publishers.

Gibbons, P. and Tehan, P. (2004). *Manipulation von Wirbelsäule.* Thorax and Becken.

Giles, L.G. and Singer, K.P. (1997). *Clinical Anatomy and Management of Low Back Pain* (Vol. 1). Elsevier Health Sciences.

Giles, L.G.F. and Singer, K.P. (2000). *The clinical anatomy and management of thoracic spine pain.* Butterworth-Heinemann.

Gouveia, L.O., Castanho, P. and Ferreira, J.J. (2009). Safety of chiropractic interventions: A systematic review. *Spine, 34*(11), E405–E413.

Greenman, P.E. (2005). *Lehrbuch der osteopathischen Medizin: mit 8 Tabellen.* Georg Thieme Verlag.

Haldeman, S., Carey, P., Townsend, M. and Papadopoulos, C. (2001). Arterial dissections following cervical manipulation: The chiropractic experience. *Canadian Medical Association Journal, 165*(7), 905–906.

Haldeman, S., Carey, P., Townsend, M. and Papadopoulos, C. (2002). Clinical perceptions of the risk of vertebral artery dissection after cervical manipulation: The effect of referral bias. *The Spine Journal, 2*(5), 334–342.

Haneline, M. and Triano, J. (2005). Cervical artery dissection. A comparison of highly dynamic mechanisms: Manipulation versus motor vehicle collision. *Journal of Manipulative and Physiological Therapeutics, 28*(1), 57–63.

Haynes, M.J. (1994). Stroke following cervical manipulation in Perth. *Chiropractic Journal of Australia, 24*, 42–46.

Henderson, D.J. (1992). Vertebral artery syndrome. In H.J. Vear (Ed.), *Chiropractic Standards of Practice and Quality of Care*. Gaithersburg, MD Aspen Publishers.

Killinger, L.Z. (2004). Chiropractic and geriatrics: A review of the training, role, and scope of chiropractic in caring for aging patients. *Clinics in Geriatric Medicine, 20*(2), 223–235.

Klougart, N., Leboeuf-Yde, C. and Rasmussen, L.R. (1996). Safety in chiropractic practice, Part I; The occurrence of cerebrovascular accidents after manipulation to the neck in Denmark from 1978–1988. *Journal of Manipulative and Physiological Therapeutics, 19*(6), 371–377.

Koss, R.W. (1990). Quality assurance monitoring of osteopathic manipulative treatment. *The Journal of the American Osteopathic Association, 90*(5), 427–434.

Liem, T. and Dobler, T.K. (2014). *Leitfaden Osteopathie: parietale techniken*. Elsevier, Urban&FischerVerlag.

Magarey, M.E., Rebbeck, T., Coughlan, B., Grimmer, K., Rivett, D.A. and Refshauge, K. (2004). Pre-manipulative testing of the cervical spine review, revision and new clinical guidelines. *Manual Therapy, 9*(2), 95–108.

Nadgir, R.N., Loevner, L.A., Ahmed, T., Moonis, G. *et al.* (2003). Simultaneous bilateral internal carotid and vertebral artery dissection following chiropractic manipulation: Case report and review of the literature. *Neuroradiology, 45*(5), 311–314.

Puentedura, E.J., March, J., Anders, J., Perez, A., Landers, M.R., Wallmann, H.W. and Cleland, J.A. (2012). Safety of cervical spine manipulation: Are adverse events preventable and are manipulations being performed appropriately? A review of 134 case reports. *Journal of Manual and Manipulative Therapy, 20*(2), 66–74.

Refshauge K.M. (2001). Do the guidelines do what they are supposed to? *Australian Journal of Physiotherapy 47*, 165–166.

Refshauge, K.M., Parry, S., Shirley, D., Larsen, D., Rivett, D.A. and Boland, R. (2002). Professional responsibility in relation to cervical spine manipulation. *Australian Journal of Physiotherapy, 48*(3), 171–179.

Rivett, D.A. and Milburn, P. (1996). A prospective study of complications of cervical spine manipulation. *Journal of Manual and Manipulative Therapy, 4*(4), 166–170.

Rivett, D.A. and Reid, D. (1998). Risk of stroke for cervical spine manipulation in New Zealand. *New Zealand Journal of Physiotherapy, 26*, 14–18.

Rivett, D.A., Thomas, L. and Bolton, B. (2005). Premanipulative testing: Where do we go from here? *New Zealand Journal of Physiotherapy, 33*(3), 78–84.

Rothwell, D.M., Bondy, S.J. and Williams, J.I. (2001). Chiropractic manipulation and stroke a population-based case-control study. *Stroke, 32*(5), 1054–1060.

Senstad, O., Leboeuf-Yde, C. and Borchgrevink, C. (1997). Frequency and characteristics of side effects of spinal manipulative therapy. *Spine, 22*(4), pp.435–440.

Shekelle, P.G., Adams, A.H., Chassin, M.R., Hurwitz, E., Phillips, R.B. and Brook, R.H. (1991). *The Appropriateness of Spinal Manipulation for Low-Back Pain*. Rand Corporation.

Stevinson, C., Honan, W., Cooke, B. and Ernst, E. (2001). Neurological complications of cervical spine manipulation. *Journal of the Royal Society of Medicine, 94*(3), 107–110.

Thanvi, B., Munshi, S.K., Dawson, S.L. and Robinson, T.G. (2005). Carotid and vertebral artery dissection syndromes. *Postgraduate Medical Journal, 81*(956), 383–388.

Triano, J. J. (2001). Biomechanics of spinal manipulative therapy. *The Spine Journal, 1*(2), 121–130.

Vickers, A. and Zollman, C. (1999). ABC of complementary medicine: the manipulative therapies: osteopathy and chiropractic. *British Medical Journal, 319*(7218), 1176.

Wainapel, S.F. and Fast, A. (2003). *Alternative Medicine and Rehabilitation: A Guide for Practitioners*. Demos Medical Publishing.

Westaway, M.D., Stratford, P. and Symons, B. (2003). False-negative extension/rotation pre-manipulative screening test on a patient with an atretic and hypoplastic vertebral artery. *Manual Therapy, 8*(2), 120–127.

World Health Organization. (2005). *WHO Guidelines on Basic Training and Safety in Chiropractic*. Geneva: World Health Organization.

# CHAPTER 5

# Pre-Manipulative Tests

## Introduction

Spinal manipulative therapy (SMT) is a therapeutic intervention that is practised across the world by health care professionals in various specialities, including osteopaths, chiropractors, physical therapists and medical doctors (Shekelle *et al.*, 1992; Rivett, Thomas and Bolton, 2005; Rubinstein *et al.*, 2011). The therapy is considered relatively safe and effective for the treatment of musculoskeletal conditions (World Health Organization, 2005). Although serious complications following the therapy are rarely reported, there have been a number of case reports of adverse events, particularly following cervical spine manipulation (Maher, 2001). To rule out the risk of an undue injury, pre-manipulative functional tests have therefore been a part of SMT for many years (Magarey *et al.*, 2004).

Over the last three decades, practitioners of SMT have adapted various protocols or clinical guidelines to detect patients at risk of complications (Thiel and Rix, 2005). These protocols are primarily developed to address all known risk factors and red flag symptoms that may contribute to serious complications (Refshauge, 2001). However, the existing pre-manipulative screening protocols have been subjected to critical reviews in recent years (Rivett *et al.*, 2005). The appropriateness, sensitivity and specificity of these protocols have been questioned due to the provocative nature of the tests, controversy surrounding the reliability and validity of the test procedures, and lack of definitive investigations supporting the protocols (Refshauge, 2001; Magarey *et al.*, 2004).

Moreover, there has been a lack of valid and reliable pre-manipulative screening tools that can accurately indicate which patients are at risk of complications from manipulative techniques (Rivett, 2001; Puentedura *et al.*, 2012). Although the current pre-manipulative testing procedures continue to be carried out in daily clinical practice, the majority of available evidence underpinning these tests is based on low-quality evidence (Cote *et al.*, 1995; Di Fabio, 1999; Licht, Christensen and Høilund-Carlsen, 2000; Westaway *et al.*, 2003). Studies of moderate level evidence, however, have failed to applaud their use (Gross and Kay, 2001). For this reason, many researchers have suggested that practitioners should emphasise on through subjective examination and sound clinical reasoning, as there is still not enough scientific evidence to show the predictive value of existing pre-manipulative tests or justify their use (Di Fabio, 1999; Licht *et al.*, 2000; Puentedura *et al.*, 2012).

The aim of this chapter is to review various pre-manipulative screening tests that are widely practised and to discuss their validity and usefulness in light of recent scientific evidence.

## Clinical Tests of the Spine

Because complications may spontaneously result from a manipulative procedure, physiotherapists/physical therapists and manipulative therapists routinely perform various pre-manipulative tests to assess patients presenting with a musculoskeletal condition. These tests are done as part of the treatment process so that SMT practitioners can identify the underlying cause(s) of a patient's presenting condition, rule out the risk of an undue injury and determine a safe and appropriate treatment plan which will increase the likelihood of a positive clinical outcome (Stude, 2005).

In general, clinical tests have one or more of five functions (see Table 5.1). They are performed to detect risk factors for a specific condition and determine the safety of the manipulative therapy (Lang and Secic, 1997). However, such tests may still be utilised when a patient is seen for preventive treatment. In this case, a given test should not aim to detect the presence or absence of specific symptoms; rather, it should be done to assess and evaluate that patient's suitability for wellness care (Stude, 2005).

**Table 5.1 Functions of clinical tests**

| Name | Characteristics |
|------|-----------------|
| Screening test | • Performed on people who are healthy and asymptomatic<br>• Has high sensitivity – that is, a good screening test is able to detect a given condition in its primary or most treatable stages<br>• Helps to identify patients with increased risk for a specific condition or disease<br>• Used to justify subsequent testing with a more specific diagnostic test<br>• Helps to determine whether direct preventive measures can be taken |
| Routine test | • Usually done on symptomatic patients as regular procedure<br>• Serves as part of a battery of tests<br>• Outcomes may be unrelated to the patient's presenting condition |
| Diagnostic test | • Performed on symptomatic subjects to revise disease probability<br>• Has high specificity<br>• Used to determine the presence or absence of a specific disorder |
| Staging test | • Done to evaluate and characterise the nature or severity of a specific condition |
| Monitoring test | • Performed to track down the gradual progress of a disease, condition or illness over time |

Sources: Lang and Secic (1997); Thiel and Rix (2005)

## Assessment and Treatment Processes

The application of SMT to the spine is associated with neurovascular and other complications (Di Fabio, 1999; Ernst, 2007; Gouveia, Castanho and Ferreira, 2009). To prevent severe complications resulting from SMT and to ensure correct patient selection, practitioners follow standard assessment methods that encompass thorough 'screening protocols' (Rivett *et al.*, 2005). Such protocols usually involve a number of processes, including a careful evaluation of the recipient's medical history, physical examination findings and provocative test results, assessment during and after treatment, and obtaining written informed consent (Magarey *et al.*, 2004; Thiel and Rix, 2005). Figure 5.1 shows a general flow chart of the assessment processes to be followed during screening examination.

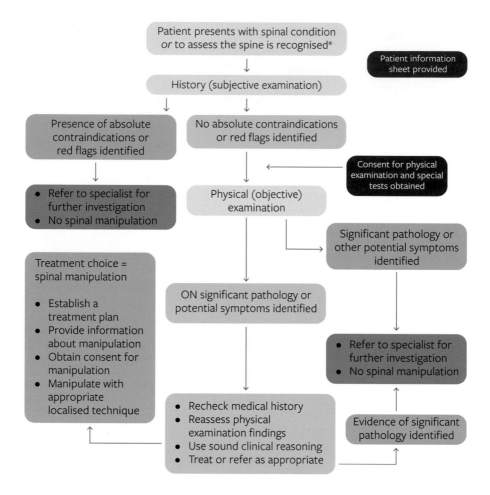

FIGURE 5.1 FLOW CHART FOR EXAMINATION OF
PATIENTS PRESENTING WITH SPINAL PROBLEM

* A need to assess the spine will be recognised if the patient has a history of trauma, fever, incontinence, unexplained weight loss, a cancer history, long-term steroid use, parenteral drug abuse, and intense localized pain and an inability to get into a comfortable position (Bratton, 1999).

## Vertebrobasilar Insufficiency Tests

Vertebrobasilar insufficiency (VBI) tests, also known as vertebral artery tests, are most commonly used for screening purposes before performing high-velocity thrust (HVT) and non-HVT manipulation (Magarey *et al.*, 2004; Childs *et al.*, 2005). These tests are provocative in nature. They are performed to test the collateral and vertebrobasilar blood supply to the brain in order to identify or recognise signs and symptoms of vertebral artery pathology, which may represent a pre-manipulation risk

(Rivett *et al.*, 2005). In addition, these tests are usually done in a clinical situation where practitioners of SMT are considering manipulation of the cervical spine as the treatment of choice (Thiel and Rix, 2005).

There have been a number of different tests to assess patients at risk of VBI, including the Barre-Lieou test, Maigne's test, Hautant's test, Underberg's test, George's cerebrovascular craniocervical functional test, the Hallpike manoeuvre, and deKleyn's test (Carey, 1995). Among these tests, deKleyn's test is one of the most commonly used. Although there are some differences in testing procedures, the general theme of all these tests is the same: extension and rotation of the head and/or neck in order to provoke cerebral ischaemia during positional change of the cervical spine (Licht *et al.*, 2000).

## Historical and Clinical Features Suggestive of VBI

- A sharp and severe non-specific, but distinct, pain – often there is no past history of a similar pain
- Pain in the head and neck – usually unilateral and sub-occipital
- A sensation of neck stiffness with or without any restriction of range of motion
- History of cervical trauma
- Limb weakness
- Ataxia/unsteadiness of gait
- Numbness – most often unilateral facial
- Nystagmus (i.e. involuntary eye movement), vestibular or cerebellar in origin
- Ipsilateral sensory abnormalities
- Hearing disturbances such as tinnitus
- Horner's syndrome
- Other neurological symptoms (e.g. ipsilateral cranial nerve abnormalities, ipsilateral limb ataxia)

Sources: Hing and Reid (2004); Thiel and Rix (2005);
Shirley, Magarey and Refshauge (2006)

### PURPOSE

VBI tests do not mimic the techniques associated with the HVT. They are intended to detect unapparent vessel pathology (e.g. dissection and/or brainstem ischaemia) by purposively compromising the blood flow into the vertebral artery (Rivett *et al.*, 2005).

### PROCEDURE

The test is usually performed in either supine lying or sitting position. The procedure involves slow passive extension and/or rotation of the recipient's head and neck to the maximum range of motion, keeping the recipient in either the supine or upright (standing or seated) position (Grant, 1996; Mitchell, 2003, 2007). The clinician sustains all positions for a minimum of ten seconds while observing for symptoms associated with VBI (Shirley *et al.*, 2006; Alshahrani, Johnson and Cordett, 2014).

### MECHANISM OF ACTION

The manoeuvre has been reported to decrease blood flow in the vertebral artery by causing a reduction of the vessel lumen, typically within the artery contralateral to the direction of rotation (Haynes and Milne, 2001; Haynes, 2002; Thiel and Rix, 2005). This compromising of vertebral artery circulation causes an ischaemia because of sudden blood loss in the brain, particularly at the pons and the medulla oblongata (Mitchell, 2007).

### POSITIVE SIGNS

In patients with VBI, the brief neurovascular event provoked by the manoeuvre often results in brainstem symptoms (Mitchell *et al.*, 2004; Shirley *et al.*, 2006). These include:

- dizziness or lightheadedness
- nausea and vomiting
- drop attacks
- temporary vision or hearing loss
- pins and needles in the tongue
- diplopia (double vision)

- pallor and sweating

- paralysis or paresis

- dysphagia and dysarthria.

If the occurrence or development of dizziness or any of the above symptoms of VBI is provoked during the manoeuvre, it has generally been considered to be a positive finding (Magee, 2008; Thiel and Rix, 2005). However, additional tests (e.g. cervical extension) should be carried out to confirm whether the provoked symptoms are potentially associated with VBI (Hing and Reid, 2004). To differentiate between symptoms related to VBI and those related to the vestibular system, the provocative VBI test should be repeated in the alternative position (Shirley *et al.*, 2006). For example, if the test procedure is performed in supine position, to confirm or differentiate the symptoms the test should be repeated in sitting position.

### AFTERCARE

If the presence of VBI becomes evident in a patient, the practitioner should immediately cease the provocative testing and return the patient's neck to the neutral position (Rivett *et al.*, 2005). In addition, because VBI is an absolute contraindication for cervical spine manipulation, manipulative procedures should be discontinued, and the patient should be referred to specialist for further medical investigation (World Health Organization, 2005; Shirley *et al.*, 2006).

## Validity of the VBI Tests

VBI tests have been thought to be an indirect technique to measure vertebral artery haemodynamics. For this reason, they are generally used to measure the degree of lumenal patency, or absence thereof, by provoking brainstem symptoms of transient ischemia (Thiel and Rix, 2005). However, the use of VBI tests as a screening tool to rule out patients at risk of cerebrovascular complications from SMT has been controversial, as reviews of literature on vertebral artery circulation studies have demonstrated varying results with regard to the effects of these tests (Grant, 1996; Rivett, Milburn and Chapple, 1998; Rivett, Sharples and Milburn, 2000; Rivett *et al.*, 2005; Di Fabio, 1999; Ernst, 2007; Puentedura *et al.*, 2012). Moreover, there have been reports of both false positive and false negative test results (Bolton, Stick and Lord, 1989; Cote *et al.*, 1995; Licht *et al.*, 1998); hence, considerable controversy exists concerning the sensitivity and specificity of these tests.

Bolton *et al.* (1989), using digital subtraction angiography, first demonstrated in a single case report that a test result might be negative, despite known occlusion of the vertebral artery. Later studies on the validity of VBI tests done by Thiel *et al.* (1994) and Licht *et al.* (1998) have suggested that these tests can also result false positive provocative findings. More recently, Haldeman, Kohlbeck and McGregor (2002) and Westaway, Stratford and Symons (2003) reported cases in which patients had VBI, but provocative screening tools, involving end-range rotation and/or extension of the head to detect the patency of the vertebral artery, did not provoke any brainstem symptoms that would contraindicate cervical spine manipulation.

In recent years, studies investigating the haemodynamic effects of cervical spine movement have employed duplex ultrasound to measure the volume, velocity or resistance to contralateral vertebral artery flow during the provocative positional manoeuvres (Licht *et al.*, 1998; Yi-Kai and Shi-Zhen, 1999; Rivett *et al.*, 2000; Haynes, 2000; Johnson *et al.*, 2000; Haynes, 2002; Mitchell, 2003; Zaina *et al.*, 2003). These studies have inconsistently demonstrated either a decrease or reduction in some of these flow parameters or no significant differences in blood flow velocity or flow rate at all, when applying pre-manipulative manoeuvres. As a result, many authors have questioned the sensitivity and positivity of the VBI tests to detect vertebral artery patency and have raised concerns about their validity to determine impedance changes to cerebrovascular circulation (Puentedura *et al.*, 2012; Rivett *et al.*, 2005; Westaway *et al.*, 2003; Rivett *et al.*, 2000; Di Fabio, 1999; Licht *et al.*, 1998; Cote *et al.*, 1995).

In contrast, Mitchell (2007) found a lot of inconsistencies in studies not finding significant reduction in vertebral artery blood flow during the provocative positional tests. Out of 20 studies reviewed, seven studies had design flaws in blood flow analyses. In addition, it was also found that only five studies measured blood flow in the fourth division of the vertebral artery and none in the third division. Therefore, it is evident that very limited research has been done to analyse the blood flow distal to the location where the resistance is believed to occur (Mitchell, 2003).

In support of the early work, Mitchell (2009) later concluded in a meta-analysis that blood flow compromise due to full or sustained contralateral rotation occurred particularly in the fourth division of the vertebral artery. Based on the review of early literature, the author also stated that sustained, full-range rotation of the cervical spine is so far the most reliable procedure to indicate the functional state of an individual's vertebrobasilar and collateral circulation.

Taken together, in light of the above discussion, it can be said that there is definitely a lack of meticulously controlled clinical trials to measure velocity changes of vertebral artery flow during sustained end-range rotation of the cervical spine. Therefore, given the inconsistencies in today's literature about the validity of VBI tests, SMT practitioners should not use those controversial results to guide evidence-based practice. Instead, they should study and appraise those findings to support the need for educated caution in pre-manipulative screening of the patients.

### Is There Any Valid Screening Tool for VBI?

There has been a lack of a reliable and valid screening tool for VBI (Childs *et al.*, 2005; Puentedura *et al.*, 2012; Alshahrani *et al.*, 2014). To date, the most reliable method to determine the functional state of a patient's collateral and vertebrobasilar circulation is the pre-manipulation provocative VBI test, particularly the sustained, full-range rotation of the cervical spine (Mitchell, 2009). Still, given the inconsistencies in current literature and the limited validity of existing VBI tests, the use of these tests have been controversial (Rivett *et al.*, 2005; Mitchell, 2007). As a result, many authors have proposed continuous-wave duplex ultrasound to assess the status of blood flow in the vertebral artery during VBI tests; however, the use of such a device has not been a practical or affordable option (Rivett, 2001; Thiel and Rix, 2005; Rivett *et al.*, 2005; Alshahrani *et al.*, 2014). As an alternative to duplex ultrasound, Haynes (2002) and Rivett (2001) suggested a simpler ultrasound device, known as the Doppler velocimeter, to indicate changes in vertebral artery blood flow during the pre-treatment VBI test. Furthermore, in a recent study, Mitchell (2009), based on a review of the literature, suggested pulsed-wave Doppler insonation with colour flow imaging as a reliable method to investigate vertebral artery blood flow during full or sustained contralateral rotation.

**Craniocervical Ligament Stability Tests**

Craniocervical ligament screening is usually performed on patients who have conditions or disorders that affect the integrity of the cervical spine ligaments, such as rheumatoid arthritis and Down syndrome, or who have suffered cervical spine trauma (i.e. hyperflexion, whiplash) (Hing and Reid, 2004). A number of tests have been advocated as part this screening, including Sharp–Purser test, anterior shear test, distraction test for the tectorial membrane, and many more. In general, these testing procedures are done prior to the application of SMT to the upper cervical spine, so that the clinician can identify any sign of upper cervical instability (Osmotherly, Rivett and Rowe, 2012).

## Potential Signs of Craniocervical Damage and Instability

- Hypermobility or empty end-feel during test movements
- Complaints of neck pain and/or headaches during sustained weight-bearing postures
- Signs of vertebral artery compromise (e.g. cerebellar ataxia)
- Catching/locking in the neck
- Paraesthesia of the lip and chin area
- Orthostatic intolerance (blood pressure drops when standing upright)
- Reproduction of symptoms of cervical instability
- Downward nystagmus (irregular eye movements)
- Poor cervical muscle strength

Sources: Hing and Reid (2004); Magee, Zachazewski and Quillen (2009)

**Table 5.2 Special tests for assessing upper cervical ligament instability**

| Test | Procedure | Positive sign | Interpretation | Validity |
|---|---|---|---|---|
| Sharp–Purser test | With the patient seated, the examiner stands at the lateral side of the patient. The patient is asked to relax the neck in a semiflexed position. The examiner places the palm of one hand on the patient's forehead, and the thumb and fingertip pads of the other hand gently hold the spinous process of the axis (C2). The patient is then asked to slowly flex the head, performing a slight cervical nod, and at the same time the examiner retracts the head in a posterior direction (Uitvlugt and Indenbaum, 1988; Mintken, Metrick and Flynn, 2008). | • A sliding motion of the head at the posterior direction in relation to the axis <br> • A 'clunk' sound <br> • Reduction in symptoms | ☐ Atlantoaxial instability | • Sensitivity: 69%; specificity: 96% (Uitvlugt and Indenbaum, 1988) |
| Anterior shear test or transverse ligament test | The patient lies supine with the head in a neutral position. The examiner stands or sits at the head of the table, supporting the occiput in the palms of the hands and 3rd–5th fingers. The examiner then places both index fingers in the space between the C2 spinous process and the occiput; thus, the index fingers are overlying the neural arch of the atlas (C1). The examiner then applies gentle pressure to the posterior arch of the atlas and lifts the head and atlas anteriorly as a unit while maintaining the head in its neutral position. This position is held for 10–20 seconds; at the same time the patient is asked to report any symptoms, excluding local pain and soreness (Mintken et al., 2008; Osmotherly et al., 2012). | • Presence of cardinal signs or symptoms <br> • Sensation of a lump in the throat | ☐ Transverse ligament insufficiency <br> ☐ Hypermobility in the atlantoaxial articulation | • A direct effect on the transverse ligament demonstrated (Osmotherly et al., 2012) |

| Test | Procedure | Positive sign | Interpretation | Validity |
|------|-----------|---------------|----------------|----------|
| Distraction test | The patient lies supine with the head relaxed on a pillow. The examiner stands or sits at the head of the couch. The examiner then gently holds the axis around its neural arch with one hand and grips the occiput with the other hand. The examiner then applies gentle distraction to the head. Normally, some movement due to a distraction force is acceptable, but this separation should not exceed 1–2mm. If symptom-free in neutral plane, the test should be repeated in slight flexion, then extension to clear membrane (Hing and Reid, 2004; Osmotherly et al., 2012). | • Excessive vertical translation when manual traction is applied<br>• Reproduction of symptoms such as nystagmus | ☐ Tectorial membrane instability<br>☐ Upper cervical ligamentous instability | • A direct effect on the tectorial membrane demonstrated (Osmotherly et al., 2012) |
| Upper cervical flexion test | The patient lies supine with the head supported by a pillow, and the examiner stands or sits at the head of the couch. The examiner holds C1 with the thumb and index finger of the sensing hand over transverse process, the web space supports the arch of the atlas, and grasps the cranium with the motive hand. The examiner then flexes the occiput using the motive hand on the cranium, while palpating for movement between the transverse process of C1 and the occiput with the sensing hand (Hing and Reid, 2004). | • Hypermobility detected with empty end-feel | ☐ Ligamentous laxity | • Sensitivity: 90%; specificity: 88% (Hall et al., 2008) |

| | | | |
|---|---|---|---|
| Lateral flexion stress test for the alar ligaments | The patient lies supine with the head supported on a pillow, and the examiner stands or sits at the head of the couch. The examiner stabilises the C2 vertebra with the thumb and index finger of the sensing hand, leaving the web space to support the spinous process, and grasps the cranium with the motive hand. The sensing hand also serves to prevent any movement occurring at the axis. The examiner then rotates the occiput, taking the atlas with it using the motive hand on the cranium. There should be 35–40 degrees of motion felt. The end-feel and the amount of motion are assessed. The test is then repeated with the upper cervical spine in flexion, neutral and extension (Beeton, 1995; Mintken et al., 2008). | • Motion available in all three positions | ☐ An alar ligament tear or arthrotic instability at the atlantoaxial joint | • A direct effect has been demonstrated (Osmotherly, Rivett and Rowe, 2013) |
| Alar ligament instability (sitting) test | With the patient in sitting position, the examiner stands at the lateral side of the patient. The examiner fixes the spinous process of C2 with the thumb and index finger of the supporting hand and grasps the cranium with the motive hand. The supporting hand should prevent any rotation occurring at the C2 segment. The examiner then side-bends the head using the motive hand or the cranium. A small (10 degrees) of side-bending should be detected with a firm end-feel (Hing and Reid, 2004). | • Greater side-bending detected | ☐ Alar ligament injury | • A direct effect has been demonstrated (Osmotherly et al., 2013) |
| Lateral stability stress test for the atlantoaxial joint | The patient lies supine with the head in a neutral position. The examiner holds the occiput and the left side of the arch of the atlas with one hand and places the other hand over the right side of the arch of the axis. The examiner then attempts to produce a lateral shear of the atlas and occiput on the axis to the right. If clear, the test is later repeated on the other side (Pettman, 1994). | • Hypermobility or reproduction of the patient's symptoms | ☐ Lateral instability to the atlantoaxial joint | • Unknown |

### Pre-Manipulative Tests of the Thoracic Spine

Unlike the cervical and lumbar regions, clinical pain syndromes associated with the thoracic region are less common. According to McKenzie and May (2006), only 5–17% of all spinal problems are thoracic in origin. In general, thoracic pain is often referred from visceral disorders, although musculoskeletal disorders of the region are common. Some major disorders of this region include kyphosis, scoliosis, ankylosing spondylitis, arthritis, juvenile kyphosis, thoracic neurofibroma, Paget's disease and tuberculosis (Ombregt, 2013).

The diagnosis and management of thoracic spine disorders have been challenging, because there has been a lack of high-quality literature for the region (Lemole *et al.*, 2002). Below are some of the special tests that are often performed to diagnose patients with thoracic spine disorders (Table 5.3).

### Pre-Manipulative Tests of the Lumbar Spine

Low back pain is a very common problem which many people experience at some stage in their lives. It is a disorder with variable etiologies. It can be caused by lumbar arthritis, spondylolisthesis, lumbar instability, spinal deformity, lumbar disc herniation, disc degeneration, spinal stenosis, painful scoliosis, lumbar injury and trapped nerves (Juniper, Le and Mladsi, 2009). Therefore, before performing SMT to the lumbar spine, it is of critical importance that the clinician accurately diagnoses the exact spinal pathology the patient is experiencing.

A number of special tests are performed as part of this screening procedure (see Table 5.4). Among these tests, the slump and the straight leg raising tests have been the most widely practised to diagnose lumbar disc herniations (Majlesi *et al.*, 2008).

**Table 5.3 Special tests for assessing serious pathology in the thoracic spine**

| Test | Procedure | Positive sign | Interpretation | Validity |
|------|-----------|---------------|----------------|----------|
| Passive rotation test | With the patient in seated position, the examiner stands in front of the patient. The examiner asks the patient to cross both arms across the chest and holds the patient's knees between his/her legs to immobilise the pelvis. The examiner then twists the patient's trunk towards the left and the right. At the end of each rotation, the examiner asks the patient to bend the head actively forwards. The examiner notes the severity of pain, range of motion and end-feel (Ombregt, 2013). | • A hard end-feel<br>• An empty end-feel with muscle spasm<br>• Increased pain during movement of the head | ☐ A hard end-feel is often suggestive of ankylosing spondylitis or advanced arthrosis<br>☐ An empty end-feel with muscle spasm suggest a severe disorder (e.g. neoplasm)<br>☐ Increased pain during movement of the head is regarded as a dural sign | • Unknown |
| Anterior-posterior rib compression test | The patient can be in either seated or standing position. The therapist stands laterally to the patient and places one hand on the anterior and another on the posterior aspects of the rib cage. The therapist compresses the rib cage by pushing the hands together and then releases the pressure (Magee, 2002). | • The rib shaft prominent in the midaxillary line<br>• Pain or point tenderness with the rib-cage compression<br>• Respiratory restrictions for both inhalation and exhalation | ☐ Possibly a rib fracture, contusion or separation | • Unknown |

| Test | Procedure | Positive sign | Interpretation | Validity |
|------|-----------|---------------|----------------|----------|
| Chest expansion test | With the patient in either seated or standing position, the examiner stands behind the patient. The examiner places his/her thumbs near to the patient's 10th ribs. The fingers of the examiner are parallel to the lateral rib cage, loosely grasping the lower hemithorax on either side of axilla. The examiner then slides his/her hands medially just sufficient to elevate a loose skin fold between the thumbs. The patient is asked to breathe and expire deeply.<br><br>Next, the examiner stands in front of the patient and places his/her thumbs laterally to each costal margin, with the hands along the lateral rib cage. The examiner then slides his/her hands medially to elevate a loose skin fold between the thumbs. The patient is asked to breathe and exhale deeply. The examiner notes the space between the thumbs in both posterior and anterior aspects and feels for the symmetry of movement of the hemithorax (Bickley and Szilagyi, 2012). | • Asymmetrical chest expansion<br>• Abnormal side expands less and lag behind the normal side | ☐ Unilateral decrease or delay in chest expansion indicates pathology on that side, such as lobar pneumonia, pleural effusion and unilateral bronchial obstruction<br>☐ Bilateral decrease in chest expansion usually suggests chronic obstructive pulmonary disease (COPD) or asthma | • Good reliability demonstrated (Sharma et al., 2004) |

| | | | |
|---|---|---|---|
| T1 nerve root stretch test | With the patient in standing position, the examiner asks the patient to lift the arm sideways from the horizontal. The patient is then asked to place the hand behind the neck by flexing the elbow (Ombregt, 2013). | • Provocation of pain between the scapulae or down the arm | ☐ Impairment of the T1 nerve root mobility | • Unknown |
| Cervical rotation lateral flexion test | With the patient in seated position, the examiner stands behind the patient. The examiner passively and maximally rotates the head away from the affected side. The examiner then attempts to laterally flex the head as far as possible, moving the ear towards the chest (Lindgren et al., 1990). | • Inability to laterally flex the head | ☐ 1st rib hypomobility in patients with brachialgia | • Reliability: Kappa = 1.0 (Flynn, Cleland and Whitman, 2008) |
| Brudzinski's sign | With the patient lying in supine, the examiner places one hand behind the patient's head and the other hand on the patient's chest. The examiner then passively flexes the patient's neck by pulling head to chest, while restraining the body from rising (Saberi and Syed, 1999). | • Involuntary flexion of the patient's hips and knees | ☐ Meningeal irritation | • Sensitivity: 5%; specificity: 95% (Thomas et al., 2002) |

**Table 5.4 Special tests for assessing serious pathology in the lumbar spine**

| Test | Procedure | Positive sign | Interpretation | Validity |
|------|-----------|---------------|----------------|----------|
| Straight leg raising test | The patient lies supine with the head and pelvis flat. The examiner slowly lifts one of the patient's legs off the table while maintaining the knee in a fully extended position. The clinician progressively continues to elevate the leg until maximum hip flexion is reached or the patient requests the examiner to stop due to pain or tightness in the back or leg. The examiner notes the angle formed between the lower limb and the examination table. In normal patients, 70–90 degrees should be possible. The same procedure is then repeated with the opposite leg (Phillips, Reider and Mehta, 2005; Magee, 2008; Majlesi et al., 2008). | • Reduced angle of hip flexion, and shooting pain radiating from the lower back down to the posterior thigh | ☐ Nerve root irritation | • Sensitivity: 52%; specificity: 89% (Majlesi et al., 2008) |
| Slump test | The patient sits on the edge of a treatment table, with legs supported, hands behind back and hips in neutral. The patient is then asked to slump, allowing the thoracic and lumbar spines to collapse into flexion while still looking straight ahead. The patient then flexes the neck by placing the chin on the chest and the examiner maintains the overpressure. The patient is then instructed to extend one knee as much as possible and at the same time the examiner dorsiflexes the ankle. The patient informs the examiner at each step during the procedure about what is being felt (Maitland, 1985; Majlesi et al., 2008). | • Reproduction of radicular pain in the back or lower limb | ☐ Increased sciatic nerve root tension | • Sensitivity: 84%; specificity: 83% (Majlesi et al., 2008) |

| | | |
|---|---|---|
| Lumbar quadrant test | This test can be performed either in the standing or seated position. In standing position, the patient stands before the examiner and extends the spine as far as possible. The examiner stabilises the ilium (largest bone of the pelvis) with one hand and grabs the shoulder with the other hand. The examiner then applies overpressure and leads the patient to extension while the patient laterally flexes and rotates to the side of pain. The examiner holds this posit on for three seconds (Baxter, 2003; Stuber *et al.*, 2014). | • Pain, numbness or tingling in the area of the back or lower limb | ☐ Localised pain is suggestive of facet syndrome<br>☐ Radiating pain into the leg indicates nerve root irritation | • Unknown |

# References

Alshahrani, A., Johnson, E.G. and Cordett, T.K. (2014). Vertebral artery testing and differential diagnosis in dizzy patients. *Physical Therapy and Rehabilitation, 1*(1), 3.

Baxter, R.E. (2003). *Pocket Guide to Musculoskeletal Assessment.* WB Saunders.

Beeton, K. (1995). Instability in the upper cervical region; clinical presentation, radiological and clinical testing. *Manipulative Physiotherapist, 27*(1), 19–32.

Bickley, L. and Szilagyi, P.G. (2012). *Bates' Guide to Physical Examination and History-Taking.* Philadelphia, PA: Lippincott Williams & Wilkins.

Bolton, P.S., Stick, P.E. and Lord, R.S. (1989). Failure of clinical tests to predict cerebral ischemia before neck manipulation. *Journal of Manipulative and Physiological Therapeutics, 12*(4), 304–307.

Bratton, R.L. (1999). Assessment and management of acute low back pain. *American Family Physician, 60*(8), 2299–2306.

Carey, P.F. (1995). A suggested protocol for the examination and treatment of the cervical spine: Managing the risk. *The Journal of the Canadian Chiropractic Association, 39*(1), 35.

Childs, J.D., Flynn, T.W., Fritz, J.M., Piva, S.R. *et al.* (2005). Screening for vertebrobasilar insufficiency in patients with neck pain: Manual therapy decision-making in the presence of uncertainty. *Journal of Orthopaedic and Sports Physical Therapy, 35*(5), 300–306.

Cote, P., Kreitz, B.G., Cassidy, J.D. and Thiel, H. (1995). The validity of the extension-rotation test as a clinical screening procedure before neck manipulation: A secondary analysis. *Journal of Manipulative and Physiological Therapeutics, 19*(3), 159–164.

Di Fabio, R.P. (1999). Manipulation of the cervical spine: Risks and benefits. *Physical Therapy, 79*(1), 50–65.

Ernst, E. (2007). Adverse effects of spinal manipulation: A systematic review. *Journal of the Royal Society of Medicine, 100*(7), 330–338.

Flynn, T.W., Cleland, J.A. and Whitman, J.M. (2008). *Users' Guide to the Musculoskeletal Examination: Fundamentals for the Evidence-Based Clinician.* Louisville, KY: Evidence in Motion.

Gouveia, L.O., Castanho, P. and Ferreira, J.J. (2009). Safety of chiropractic interventions: A systematic review. *Spine, 34*(11), E405–E413.

Grant, R. (1996). Vertebral artery testing: The Australian Physiotherapy Association Protocol after 6 years. *Manual Therapy, 1*(3), 149–153.

Gross, A.R. and Kay, T.M. (2001). Guidelines for pre-manipulative testing of the cervical spine-an appraisal. *Australian Journal of Physiotherapy, 47*(3), 166–167.

Haldeman, S., Kohlbeck, F.J. and McGregor, M. (2002). Unpredictability of cerebrovascular ischemia associated with cervical spine manipulation therapy: A review of sixty-four cases after cervical spine manipulation. *Spine, 27*(1), 49–55.

Hall, T.M., Robinson, K.W., Fujinawa, O., Akasaka, K. and Pyne, E.A. (2008). Intertester reliability and diagnostic validity of the cervical flexion-rotation test. *Journal of Manipulative and Physiological Therapeutics, 31*(4), 293–300.

Haynes, M.J. and Milne, N. (2001). Color duplex sonographic findings in human vertebral arteries during cervical rotation. *Journal of Clinical Ultrasound, 29*(1), 14–24.

Haynes, M.J. (2000). Vertebral arteries and neck rotation: Doppler velocimeter and duplex results compared. *Ultrasound in Medicine and Biology, 26*(1), 57–62.

Haynes, M.J. (2002). Vertebral arteries and cervical movement: Doppler ultrasound velocimetry for screening before manipulation. *Journal of Manipulative and Physiological Therapeutics, 25*(9), 556–567.

Haynes, M.J. (2002). Vertebral arteries and cervical movement: Doppler ultrasound velocimetry for screening before manipulation. *Journal of Manipulative and Physiological Therapeutics, 25*(9), 556–567.

Hing, W. and Reid, D. (2004). *Cervical Spine Management: Pre-Screening Requirement for New Zealand*. Auckland: New Zealand Manipulative Physiotherapists Association.

Johnson, C., Grant, R., Dansie, B., Taylor, J. and Spyropolous, P. (2000). Measurement of blood flow in the vertebral artery using colour duplex Doppler ultrasound: Establishment of the reliability of selected parameters. *Manual Therapy, 5*(1), 21–29.

Juniper, M., Le, T.K. and Mladsi, D. (2009). The epidemiology, economic burden, and pharmacological treatment of chronic low back pain in France, Germany, Italy, Spain and the UK: A literature-based review. *Expert Opinion on Pharmacotherapy, 10*(16), 2581–2592.

Lang, T.A. and Secic, M. (1997). *How to Report Statistics in Medicine*. Philadelphia, PA: American College of Physicians.

Lemole, G.M., Bartolomei, J., Henn, J.S. and Sonntag, V.K.H. (2002). Thoracic fractures. In A.R. Vaccaro (Ed.), *Fractures of the Cervical, Thoracic, and Lumbar Spine*. Boca Raton, FL: CRC Press.

Licht, P.B., Christensen, H.W. and Høilund-Carlsen, P.F. (2000). Is there a role for premanipulative testing before cervical manipulation? *Journal of Manipulative and Physiological Therapeutics, 23*(3), 175–179.

Licht, P.B., Christensen, H.W., Højgaard, P. and Høilund-Carlsen, P.F. (1998). Triplex ultrasound of vertebral artery flow during cervical rotation. *Journal of Manipulative and Physiological Therapeutics, 21*(1), 27–31.

Lindgren, K.A., Leino, E., Hakola, M. and Hamberg, J. (1990). Cervical spine rotation and lateral flexion combined motion in the examination of the thoracic outlet. *Archives of Physical Medicine and Rehabilitation, 71*(5), 343–344.

Magarey, M.E., Rebbeck, T., Coughlan, B., Grimmer, K., Rivett, D.A. and Refshauge, K. (2004). Pre-manipulative testing of the cervical spine review, revision and new clinical guidelines. *Manual Therapy, 9*(2), 95–108.

Magee, D.J. (2002). *Orthopedic Physical Assessment*, 4th edition. St Louis, MO: Elsevier Health Sciences.

Magee, D.J. (2008). *Orthopedic Physical Assessment*, 5th edition. St Louis, MO: Elsevier Health Sciences.

Magee, D.J., Zachazewski, J.E. and Quillen, W.S. (2009). Cervical spine. In: *Pathology and Intervention in Musculoskeletal Rehabilitation*. St Louis, MO: Saunders Elsevier.

Maher, C. (2001). AJP forum: Pre-manipulative testing of the cervical spine. *Australian Journal of Physiotherapy, 47*(3), 163–164.

Maitland, G.D. (1985). The slump test: Examination and treatment. *Australian Journal of Physiotherapy, 31*(6), 215–219.

Majlesi, J., Togay, H., Ünalan, H. and Toprak, S. (2008). The sensitivity and specificity of the slump and the straight leg raising tests in patients with lumbar disc herniation. *Journal of Clinical Rheumatology, 14*(2), 87–91.

McKenzie, R. and May, S. (2006). *The Cervical and Thoracic Spine: Mechanical Diagnosis and Therapy*. Windham, NH: Orthopedic Physical Therapy Products.

Mintken, P.E., Metrick, L. and Flynn, T. (2008). Upper cervical ligament testing in a patient with os odontoideum presenting with headaches. *Journal of Orthopaedic and Sports Physical Therapy, 38*(8), 465–475.

Mitchell, J. (2007). Doppler insonation of vertebral artery blood flow changes associated with cervical spine rotation: Implications for manual therapists. *Physiotherapy Theory and Practice, 23*(6), 303–313.

Mitchell, J. (2009). Vertebral artery blood flow velocity changes associated with cervical spine rotation: A meta-analysis of the evidence with implications for professional practice. *Journal of Manual and Manipulative Therapy, 17*(1), 46–57.

Mitchell, J., Keene, D., Dyson, C., Harvey, L., Pruvey, C. and Phillips, R. (2004). Is cervical spine rotation, as used in the standard vertebrobasilar insufficiency test, associated with a measureable change in intracranial vertebral artery blood flow? *Manual Therapy, 9*(4), 220–227.

Mitchell, J.A. (2003). Changes in vertebral artery blood flow following normal rotation of the cervical spine. *Journal of Manipulative and Physiological Therapeutics, 26*(6), 347–351.

Ombregt, L. (2013). *Clinical Examination of the Thoracic Spine: A System of Orthopaedic Medicine*. St Louis, MO: Elsevier Health Sciences.

Osmotherly, P.G., Rivett, D. and Rowe, L.J. (2013). Toward understanding normal craniocervical rotation occurring during the rotation stress test for the alar ligaments. *Physical Therapy, 93*(7), 986–992.

Osmotherly, P.G., Rivett, D.A. and Rowe, L.J. (2012). The anterior shear and distraction tests for craniocervical instability: An evaluation using magnetic resonance imaging. *Manual Therapy, 17*(5), 416–421.

Pettman, E. (1994). Stress tests of the craniovertebral joints. In: *Grieve's Modern Manual Therapy: The Vertebral Column*, 2nd edition. Edinburgh: Churchill Livingstone.

Phillips, F.M., Reider, B. and Mehta, V. (2005). Lumbar spine. In B. Reider (Ed.), *The Orthopaedic Physical Examination*, 2nd edition. Philadelphia, PA: Elsevier Saunders.

Puentedura, E.J., March, J., Anders, J., Perez, A. *et al.* (2012). Safety of cervical spine manipulation: Are adverse events preventable and are manipulations being performed appropriately? A review of 134 case reports. *Journal of Manual and Manipulative Therapy, 20*(2), 66–74.

Refshauge, K. (2001). Do the guidelines do what they are supposed to? *Australian Journal of Physiotherapy, 47*(3), 165–166.

Rivett D., Sharples K. and Milburn P. (2000). Vertebral artery blood flow during pre-manipulative testing of the cervical spine. In K.P. Singer (Ed.), *Proceedings of the International Federation of Orthopaedic and Manipulative Therapists Conference*. Perth: International Federation of Orthopaedic and Manipulative Therapists.

Rivett, D.A. (2001). A valid pre-manipulative screening tool is needed. *Australian Journal of Physiotherapy, 47*(3), 166.

Rivett, D.A., Milburn, P.D. and Chapple, C. (1998). Negative pre-manipulative vertebral artery testing despite complete occlusion: A case of false negativity? *Manual Therapy, 3*(2), 102–107.

Rivett, D.A., Thomas, L. and Bolton, B. (2005). Premanipulative testing: Where do we go from here? *New Zealand Journal of Physiotherapy, 33*(3), 78–84.

Rubinstein, S.M., van Middelkoop, M., Assendelft, W.J., de Boer, M.R. and van Tulder, M.W. (2011). Spinal manipulative therapy for chronic low-back pain. *Cochrane Database of Systematic Reviews, 16*(2).

Saberi, A. and Syed, S.A. (1999). Meningeal signs: Kernig's sign and Brudzinski's sign. *Hospital Physician, 35*, 23–26.

Sharma, J., Senjyu, H., Williams, L. and White, C. (2004). Intra-tester and inter-tester reliability of chest expansion measurement in clients with ankylosing spondylitis and healthy individuals. *Journal of the Japanese Physical Therapy Association, 7*(1), 23.

Shekelle, P.G., Adams, A.H., Chassin, M.R., Hurwitz, E.L. and Brook, R.H. (1992). Spinal manipulation for low-back pain. *Annals of Internal Medicine, 117*(7), 590–598.

Shirley, D., Magarey, M. and Refshauge, K. (2006). *Clinical Guidelines for Assessing Vertebrobasilar Insufficiency in the Management of Cervical Spine Disorders.* Australian Physiotherapy Association.

Stuber, K., Lerede, C., Kristmanson, K., Sajko, S. and Bruno, P. (2014). The diagnostic accuracy of the Kemp's test: A systematic review. *The Journal of the Canadian Chiropractic Association, 58*(3), 258.

Stude, D.E. (2005). A functional pre-manipulative spinal orthopedic assessment maneuver. *Journal of Chiropractic Medicine, 4*(2), 61–69.

Thiel, H. and Rix, G. (2005). Is it time to stop functional pre-manipulation testing of the cervical spine? *Manual Therapy, 10*(2), 154–158.

Thiel, H., Wallace, K., Donat, J. and Yong-Hing, K. (1994). Effect of various head and neck positions on vertebral artery blood flow. *Clinical Biomechanics, 9*(2), 105–110.

Thomas, K.E., Hasbun, R., Jekel, J. and Quagliarello, V.J. (2002). The diagnostic accuracy of Kernig's sign, Brudzinski's sign, and nuchal rigidity in adults with suspected meningitis. *Clinical Infectious Diseases, 35*(1), 46–52.

Uitvlugt, G. and Indenbaum, S. (1988). Clinical assessment of atlantoaxial instability using the sharp-purser test. *Arthritis and Rheumatism, 31*(7), 918–922.

Westaway, M.D., Stratford, P. and Symons, B. (2003). False-negative extension/rotation pre-manipulative screening test on a patient with an atretic and hypoplastic vertebral artery. *Manual Therapy, 8*(2), 120–127.

World Health Organization. (2005). *WHO Guidelines on Basic Training and Safety in Chiropractic.* Geneva: World Health Organization.

Yi-Kai, L. and Shi-Zhen, Z. (1999). Changes and implications of blood flow velocity of the vertebral artery during rotation and extension of the head. *Journal of Manipulative and Physiological Therapeutics, 22*(2), 91–95.

Zaina, C., Grant, R., Johnson, C., Dansie, B., Taylor, J. and Spyropolous, P. (2003). The effect of cervical rotation on blood flow in the contralateral vertebral artery. *Manual Therapy, 8*(2), 103–109.

# CHAPTER 6

# Safety of Spinal Manipulation in the Treatment of Lumbar Disc Pathology

## Current Concepts in Literature: Review 2016
*Dr James Inklebarger*

## Introduction

Spinal manipulation is considered a relatively risk-free intervention for the treatment of musculoskeletal conditions when administered skilfully and accurately. The primary adverse reactions include temporary exacerbation of symptoms or new local symptoms. Serious complications of manipulation are rarely reported. However, in recent years, a number of adverse outcomes associated with lumbar spine manipulation, such as lumbar disc annular tears (LDAT), lumbar disc herniation (LDH) and degenerative disc disease (DDD), have been reported in the literature (Boucher and Robidoux, 2014). In contrast, there is also a growing body of evidence that spinal manipulation (SMT) is a safe and effective intervention for the management of acute and chronic discogenic low back pain (DLBP) (Oliphant, 2004).

It is, therefore, important to determine whether the risks associated with SMT can outweigh the benefits. Informed consent and modern clinical decision-making processes rely on the evidence base of medicine to calculate risk versus benefit ratios. The methodology can also be applied to SMT for the management of DLBP. The actual risk of serious complications, such as cauda equina syndrome (CES), LDAT and LDH, arising from lumbar manipulation can be ascertained by reviewing literature reporting adverse outcomes.

Although determining an actual risk versus benefit ratio for SMT is profoundly difficult on a global scale, the job is less strenuous when it is calculated in a selected group of people. As chiropractors in the United States represent the largest professional body of lumbar spine manipulators across the globe (Weeks, 2009), the total number of reported complications following SMT from this group can be used to determine an estimated risk associated with the therapy. However, it is fair to point out that these reports appear to have lumped chiropractors together with other spinal manipulators, such as surgeons, physiotherapists and massage therapists, as well as unskilled lay and general practitioners who may have less skill, education and experience.

## Risk v Benefit Ratio for Lumbar SMT

The risk of serious complications after lumbar SMT can be estimated by excluding the minor and transient adverse reactions. This can be accomplished by making a statistical comparison between the number of serious adverse events reported in the literature and the numbers of patients receiving SMT. Many authors, including Adams and Sim (1998), Cagnie et al. (2004) and Smith et al. (1995), have attempted to put things in perspective. However, the exact rate of such adverse events is yet not known. Moreover, these estimates of risks have been reported to vary widely between studies (see Table 6.1).

**Table 6.1 Rate of serious adverse events due to lumbar manipulation**

| Rate of complications | Nature of complication | Authors |
| --- | --- | --- |
| 1 per 10–100 million | CES | Shekelle et al. (1992) |
| 1 per 286 million | CES | Haldeman and Rubinstein (1992) |
| 1 per 1 million | CES | Assendelft, Boulter and Knipschild (1996) |
| 1 per 100 million | CES | Coulter (1998) |
| 1 per 3.7 million | LDH, LDAT and CES | Oliphant (2004) |

The rate of serious complications after lumbar manipulation, such as LDH, LDAT and CES, have been reported in the chiropractic literature as 1 per 3.7 million (Oliphant, 2004), with the risk virtually doubling in cases where lumbar SMT was performed under anaesthesia (MUA) (Haldeman and Rubenstein, 1992). Using 40 years of United States chiropractic patient data, Oliphant calculated the occurrence of LDH/CES in patients complaining of DLBP to be 1 in 46 million (Oliphant, 2004). In contrast to this study, Haldeman and Rubinstein (1992) in an earlier study have estimated SMT-associated CES to be 1 per 286 million.

To put the relative safety of manipulation in a clearer perspective, some authors have compared the safety of lumbar SMT against the conventional therapies such as non-steroidal anti-inflammatory drugs (NSAIDs) and lumbar spine fusion (LSF). NSAIDs are known to have serious renal, gastrointestinal (gastric erosions/ulcers leading to death) and asthma-exacerbating side effects. Coulter (1998) suggests that the use of lumbar manipulation is far safer than NSAIDs, as NSAIDs are associated with 3.2 complications per 1000 patients. Furthermore, excluding some of the serious adverse effects of NSAIDs such as renal complications and asthma symptom exacerbations, Henry *et al.* (1993, 1996) reported that the rate of NSAIDs-associated upper gastrointestinal complications in the adult population was 147 per 100,000 patients.

LSF is a popular surgical method for the management of intractable DLBP. Over 400,000 Americans undergo this costly procedure every year. Unfortunately, LSF is associated with many complications and had a failure rate of 13.2% in a five-year follow-up (Greiner-Perth *et al.*, 2004). Despite the high failure rate of LSF, many patients suffering severe intractable discogenic pain have reported high levels of surgical satisfaction after the procedure. Nevertheless, LSF and surgical alternatives such as artificial disc replacement are permanent life-altering interventions, and therefore should be reserved for those whose conditions have failed to improve following conservative treatment (Inklebarger, 2014).

Taken together, it can be said that the risk of serious complications due to lumbar SMT is very low. Although some case-report authors would argue otherwise (Malawski *et al.*, 1993; Li, 1989), based on the findings in the recent literature, SMT appears to be very safe for the treatment of low back pain (LBP). In fact, SMT has repeatedly been recommended as a relatively safe and effective intervention for the management of lumbar disc diseases.

For example, Bronfort *et al.* (2004) in a systematic review found SMT as effective as medical care for both the short- and long-term relief of LBP-associated disc herniation. Some studies even reported high-velocity, low-amplitude thrust (HVLAT) techniques as safe procedures for expediting the recovery period of both acute and chronic LDH (Quon *et al.*, 1989; Leemann *et al.*, 2014).

Biomedical research utilises a more novel approach to determine adverse effects of a therapy. Not surprisingly, the safety of SMT is also ensured by damage markers analysis. In a randomised controlled trial, Achalandabaso *et al.* (2014) recently explored the possibility of soft-tissue damage following SMT, analysing the elevation of acute phase proteins and inflammatory biomarkers. The authors found no significant changes in any of the studied tissue damage markers and suggested SMT to be innocuous to the joints and surrounding tissues.

In comparison with other common treatments such as NSAIDs and surgery, it has also been demonstrated that SMT is comparatively far safer than those therapies for LBP management. However, the use of gentle SMT technique instead of rotatory thrust technique has strongly been suggested to further reduce the risk of an undue adverse event (Haldeman, Chapman-Smith and Petersen, 2004).

## Is Lumbar SMT Associated with Lumbar Disc Pathology?

The pathogenetic relationship between the onset of lumbar pathologies and the application of lumbar manipulation has yet not been demonstrated. In fact, many authors have questioned the validity of such a relationship, because so far only a few cases have been reported. In addition, most of these reports are poorly documented and very old (Tamburrelli, Genitiempo and Logroscino, 2011). The authors also stated that such a cause–effect relationship was merely assumed from a temporary onset of symptoms after SMT.

In the literature, SMT is often described as an extremely rare cause of CES. Because CES can occur spontaneously in the absence of SMT, a pathogenetic relationship between CES and SMT may be invalid. In fact, CES is usually associated with a large LDH and may be complicated by some other lumbar conditions such as congenital canal stenosis and spondylolisthesis. Risk factors of CES include obesity, male gender, history of back disorders, greater than 40 years of age and a history of occupational or sporting activity that involves repetitive spinal loading (Kostova and Koleva, 2001).

In laboratory spinal testing, it has been demonstrated that a combination of hyperflexion, lateral bending and severe compression can result in annular tear and disc prolapse (Adams and Hutton, 1982). However, for disc prolapse to occur, both an annular tear (fissure) and a fragment within the disc must be present (Brinckmann and Porter, 1994). The combination of spinal movements that causes LDH often occurs during heavy lifting. Epidemiological studies also suggest that people engaged in combined repetitive lifting with twisting motions are three times more likely to suffer LDH (Kelsey et al., 1984).

LDH can occur in teen and adolescent populations with non-specific LBP (Kumar et al., 2007; Dang and Liu, 2010). Although the pathogenetic processes are not yet known, this may be caused by daily school activities (Kaspiris et al., 2010). Furthermore, there is evidence that the healthy or mildly degenerated disc is more prone to disc herniation than the severely degenerated or arthritic spine (Schmidt et al., 2007a, 2007b). Taken together, it can be hypothesised that for SMT to exacerbate symptoms of LDH or CES, the disc must already be fragmented and fissured. Therefore, it is reasonable to conclude that LDH also occurs in the absence of manipulation.

It is also essential to consider the fact that as many as 40% of the patients attending chiropractors may have existing DLBP (Schwarzer et al., 1995). Besides, a number of studies have demonstrated that disc degeneration is strongly associated with hereditary predisposition (Battie et al., 1995a, 1995b; Matsui et al., 1998; Sambrook, MacGregor and Spector, 1999). It therefore becomes more evident that the risk of serious discogenic complications associated with SMT is extremely rare, although alleged exacerbation and causation of DLBP are the most common causes of malpractice claims against chiropractors (Jagbandhansingh, 1997).

In light of the above discussion, it can be presumed that practitioners in most cases do not cause the undue injury but aggravate a pre-existing lesion for which they are consulted, although one may also speculate that at least some of the SMT-attributed cases could have had the same onset and outcome independently. However, the fact is when a clinician administers SMT during the prodrome of a disc herniation, he/she actually puts himself/herself at risk of being identified as the cause, if leg pain and neurological deficit ensue. For example, clinicians who perform grade 5 side-postural SMT in a patient presenting with acute LDH may find themselves blamed from a medico-legal standpoint if symptoms flare during the prodrome of acute disc herniation.

Therefore, the complications associated with SMT can be attributed to poor clinical judgement, inadequate skill or inappropriate use of techniques. For this reason, to reduce the risk of an undue injury, it is of critical importance that sound clinical reasoning is practised, adequate skill is exercised and quality care is provided. Some SMT practitioners thus advocate gentler manual flexion-distraction techniques such as Barnes and Cox as a more cautious approach to DLBP management.

## Conclusion

From the above discussion, it can be concluded that lumbar manipulation is a relatively safe and effective intervention for the management of DLBP. The frequency of serious adverse events due to SMT, such as a clinically worsened disc herniation or CES in a patient presenting with LDH, is very low. In fact, the cause-and-effect relationship between lumbar SMT and serious lumbar pathologies is yet not established. Perhaps SMT does not cause lumbar disc pathologies but merely worsens a pre-existing condition. Therefore, to avoid the risk of an undue injury, it is of significant importance that a careful pre-manipulative assessment is conducted. In addition, greater care should be taken while determining the appropriateness of a manipulation technique before applying it to a patient.

However, more research is needed to accurately determine the incidence of disc injury or increased disc symptoms following SMT. Studies researching on this should develop and apply adequate experimental approaches to identify whether SMT can actually cause a disc herniation. Furthermore, it is essential that more high-quality research is done on SMT, so that the benefit of spinal manipulation in the treatment of LDH can be compared with other conservative treatments, and it can be determined which patient group would benefit most from which type of treatment.

## Summary

- The frequency of SMT-associated LDH, LDAT or CES is very low – 1 per 37 million manipulations.

- LDH, LDAT and CES have a strong genetic component, often occur spontaneously and may have a natural history of evolution independent of lumbar SMT. Appropriate diagnosis of pre-existing and presenting condition, thorough physical examination and accurate record keeping are therefore recommended to avoid potential temporal associations.

- Lumbar spine flexion should be avoided when performing rotational lumbar SMT techniques.

- Grade 5 rotary or high-velocity thrust (HVT) manipulations performed in acute DLBP or in cases of non-contained bulge or sequestercd LDH may have medico-legal consequences. Therefore, they should be avoided.

- Use of gentle, long-axis stationary and manual traction techniques such as Cox, Leander and McManis, with usual precautions, may represent more conservative management options.

- Feedback from an alert and awake patient enhances safety. Because lumbar MUA increases the risk of serious SMT complications, it should therefore be avoided.

# References

Achalandabaso, A., Plaza-Manzano, G., Lomas-Vega, R., Martínez-Amat, A. *et al.* (2014). Tissue damage markers after a spinal manipulation in healthy subjects: A preliminary report of a randomized controlled trial. *Disease Markers*, Epub.

Adams, G. and Sim, J. (1998). A survey of UK manual therapists' practice of and attitudes towards manipulation and its complications. *Physiotherapy Research International, 3*(3), 206–227.

Adams, M.A. and Hutton, W.C. (1982). Prolapsed intervertebral disc: A hyperflexion injury. *Spine, 7*(3), 184–191.

Assendelft, V.J., Bouter, L.M. and Knipschild, P.G. (1996). Complications of spinal manipulation. *Journal of Family Practice, 42*(5), 475–480.

Battie, M.C., Haynor, D.R., Fisher, L.D., Gill, K., Gibbons, L.E. and Videman, T. (1995a). Similarities in degenerative findings on magnetic resonance images of the lumbar spines of identical twins. *Journal of Bone and Joint Surgery, 77*(11), 1662–1670.

Battie, M.C., Videman, T., Gibbons, L.E., Fisher, L.D., Manninen, H. and Gill, K. (1995b). Determinants of lumbar disc degeneration: A study relating lifetime exposures and magnetic resonance imaging findings in identical twins. *Spine, 20*(24), 2601–2612.

Boucher, P. and Robidoux, S. (2014). Lumbar disc herniation and cauda equina syndrome following spinal manipulative therapy. A review of six court decisions in Canada. *Journal of Forensic and Legal Medicine, 22*, 159–169.

Brinckmann, P. and Porter, R.W. (1994). A laboratory model of lumbar disc protrusion: Fissure and fragment. *Spine, 19*(2), 228–235.

Bronfort, G., Haas, M., Evans, R.L. and Bouter, L.M. (2004). Efficacy of spinal manipulation and mobilization for low back pain and neck pain: A systematic review and best evidence synthesis. *The Spine Journal, 4*(3), 335–356.

Cagnie, B., Vinck, E., Beernaert, A. and Cambier, D. (2004). How common are side effects of spinal manipulation and can these side effects be predicted? *Manual Therapy, 9*(3), 151–156.

Coulter, I.D. (1998). Efficacy and risks of chiropractic manipulation: What does the evidence suggest? *Integrative Medicine, 1*(2), 61–66.

Dang, L. and Liu, Z. (2010). A review of current treatment for lumbar disc herniation in children and adolescents. *European Spine Journal, 19*(2), 205.

Greiner-Perth, R., Boehm, H., Allam, Y., Elsaghir, H. and Franke, J. (2004). Reoperation rate after instrumented posterior lumbar interbody fusion: A report on 1680 cases. *Spine, 29*(22), 2516–2520.

Haldeman, S. and Rubinstein, S.M. (1992). Cauda equina syndrome in patients undergoing manipulation of the lumbar spine. *Spine, 17*(12), 1469–1473.

Haldeman, S., Chapman-Smith, D. and Petersen, D.M. (2004). *Guidelines for Chiropractic Quality Assurance and Practice Parameters: Proceedings of the Mercy Center Consensus Conference.* Burlington, MA: Jones & Bartlett Learning.

Henry, D., Dobson, A. and Turner, C. (1993). Variability in the risk of major gastrointestinal complications from nonaspirin nonsteroidal anti-inflammatory drugs. *Gastroenterology, 105*, 1078–1078.

Henry, D., Lim, L.L., Rodriguez, L.A.G., Gutthann, S.P. *et al*. S. (1996). Variability in risk of gastrointestinal complications with individual non-steroidal anti-inflammatory drugs: Results of a collaborative meta-analysis. *British Medical Journal, 312*(7046), 1563–1566.

Inklebarger, J. (2014). Discogenic lower back pain: Current concepts. *International Musculoskeletal Medicine, 36*(2), 50–53.

Jagbandhansingh, M.P. (1997). Most common causes of chiropractic malpractice lawsuits. *Journal of Manipulative and Physiological Therapeutics, 20*(1), 60–64.

Kaspiris, A., Grivas, T.B., Zafiropoulou, C., Vasiliadis, E. and Tsadira, O. (2010). Nonspecific low back pain during childhood: A retrospective epidemiological study of risk factors. *Journal of Clinical Rheumatology, 16*(2), 55–60.

Kelsey, J.L., Githens, P.B., White, A.A., Holford, T.R. *et al*. (1984). An epidemiologic study of lifting and twisting on the job and risk for acute prolapsed lumbar intervertebral disc. *Journal of Orthopaedic Research, 2*(1), 61–66.

Kostova, V. and Koleva, M. (2001). Back disorders (low back pain, cervicobrachial and lumbosacral radicular syndromes) and some related risk factors. *Journal of the Neurological Sciences, 192*(1), 17–25.

Kumar, R., Kumar, V., Das, N.K., Behari, S. and Mahapatra, A.K. (2007). Adolescent lumbar disc disease: Findings and outcome. *Child's Nervous System, 23*(11), 1295–1299.

Leemann, S., Peterson, C.K., Schmid, C., Anklin, B. and Humphreys, B.K. (2014). Outcomes of acute and chronic patients with magnetic resonance imaging–confirmed symptomatic lumbar disc herniations receiving high-velocity, low-amplitude, spinal manipulative therapy: A prospective observational cohort study with one-year follow-up. *Journal of Manipulative and Physiological Therapeutics, 37*(3), 155–163.

Li, J.S. (1989). Acute rupture of lumbar intervertebral disc caused by violent manipulation. *Zhonghua wai ke za zhi [Chinese Journal of Surgery], 27*(8), 477.

Malawski, S., Milecki, M., Nowak-Misiak, M., Sokólski, B. and Szlapin, M. (1993). Complications of vertebral disc and spinal diseases after manipulation therapy. *Chirurgia narzadów ruchu i ortopedia polska, 58*(2), 3.

Matsui, H., Kanamori, M., Ishihara, H., Yudoh, K., Naruse, Y. and Tsuji, H. (1998). Familial predisposition for lumbar degenerative disc disease: A case-control study. *Spine, 23*(9), 1029–1034.

Oliphant, D. (2004). Safety of spinal manipulation in the treatment of lumbar disk herniations: A systematic review and risk assessment. *Journal of Manipulative and Physiological Therapeutics, 27*(3), 197–210.

Quon, J.A., Cassidy, J.D., O'Connor, S.M. and Kirkaldy-Willis, W.H. (1989). Lumbar intervertebral disc herniation: Treatment by rotational manipulation. *Journal of Manipulative and Physiological Therapeutics, 12*(3), 220–227.

Sambrook, P.N., MacGregor, A.J. and Spector, T.D. (1999). Genetic influences on cervical and lumbar disc degeneration. *Arthritis and Rheumatology, 42*(2), 336.

Schmidt, H., Kettler, A., Heuer, F., Simon, U., Claes, L. and Wilke, H.J. (2007a). Intradiscal pressure, shear strain, and fiber strain in the intervertebral disc under combined loading. *Spine, 32*(7), 748–755.

Schmidt, H., Kettler, A., Rohlmann, A., Claes, L. and Wilke, H.J. (2007b). The risk of disc prolapses with complex loading in different degrees of disc degeneration: A finite element analysis. *Clinical Biomechanics, 22*(9), 988–998.

Schwarzer, A.C., Aprill, C.N., Derby, R., Fortin, J., Kine, G. and Bogduk, N. (1995). The prevalence and clinical features of internal disc disruption in patients with chronic low back pain. *Spine, 20*(17), 1878–1883.

Shekelle, P.G., Adams, A.H., Chassin, M.R., Hurwitz, E.L. and Brook, R.H. (1992). Spinal manipulation for low-back pain. *Annals of Internal Medicine, 117*(7), 590–598.

Smith, S.E., Darden, B.V., Rhyne, A.L. and Wood, K.E. (1995). Outcome of unoperated discogram-positive low back pain. *Spine, 20*(18), 1997.

Tamburrelli, F.C., Genitiempo, M. and Logroscino, C.A. (2011). Cauda equina syndrome and spine manipulation: Case report and review of the literature. *European Spine Journal, 20*(1), 128–131.

Weeks, W.B. (2009). The supply and demand of chiropractors in the United States from 1996 to 2005. *Alternative Therapies in Health and Medicine, 15*(3), 36.

# CHAPTER 7

# Clinical Presentation of Vertebral Artery Dissection

*Dr James Inklebarger*

Vertebral artery dissection (VAD) is a tear in the wall of the vertebral artery located in the neck. This often causes an interruption of blood flow within the layers of the arterial wall, ultimately resulting in a blood clot in the artery.

## Epidemiology

The overall incidence of VAD is relatively rare – roughly 1–1.5 per 100,000 (Park *et al.*, 2008). Kim and Schulman (2009), reviewing a number of population-based studies, suggested that the average annual incidence of VAD in the United States and France was 1–1.1 per 100,000. Surprisingly, the authors also found that from 1994 to 2003, the rate of VAD incidences gradually increased approximately threefold. However, this surge in incidence rate has been attributed to the gradual increase of more sophisticated diagnostic device use such as MRI in clinical practice.

## Clinical Presentation

VAD is an increasingly acknowledged cause of brainstem stroke, especially in young and otherwise healthy adults under 45 years of age. In patients with VAD, the typical presentation includes severe pain in the back of the head and neck, with a recent history of injury in either of those two areas. These patients subsequently develop focal neurological deficits as a result of the brainstem or cerebellum ischaemia. The signs of a neurologic deficit may not show up unless a latent period as long as three days is passed. However, it has been reported that the symptoms can even take weeks or years to appear. Many patients present only at the onset of neurological symptoms (Fukuhara *et al.*, 2015).

In general, headache may be the only presenting symptom of VAD. Kim and Schulman (2009) found that in 50–75% of cases a headache was present with almost half of patients reporting a completely unique type of pain, which they had never experienced before. In addition, in 40% of cases an occurrence of trauma has been reported days or weeks preceding the dissection; however, the trauma has been found to be minor 90% of the time (Debette, 2014). More than 75% of VAD patients recover completely or are left with minimal residual dysfunction. The remainder often develop a severe disability, although the mortality rate is rare – about 2% (Campos-Herrera *et al.*, 2008).

## Is Spinal Manipulation Associated with VAD?

Cervical spine manipulation (CSM) has been reported to be associated with VAD. This has been thought to result from over-stretching of the artery during rotational thrust manipulation (Nadgir *et al.*, 2003), and dissection of the arteries has been presumed to occur at the level of the atlantoaxial joint. The incidence of VAD due to CSM, however, is considered to be rare. The calculated rate of incidence is 1 per 5.85 million cervical manipulations (Haldeman *et al.*, 2002). Moreover, so far there is no conclusive evidence that supports a strong association between neck manipulation and stroke (Haynes *et al.*, 2012).

Nevertheless, the risk of a vascular accident is not negligible; therefore, appropriate precautions should be taken to prevent the risk of VAD causation and/or exacerbation following CSM. The World Health Organization (2005) guidelines have defined a number of absolute to relative contraindications and red flag symptoms in which manipulation should never be performed. These include long-term anticoagulant therapy, certain blood dyscrasias, collagen diseases, congenital malformations and a prior history of a cerebrovascular accident. In addition, Vautravers and Maigne (1999) have made five recommendations to restrict the use of rotational thrust CSM in potentially at-risk populations. The French Society of Orthopaedic and Osteopathic Manual Medicine (SOFMMOO) later adopted these recommendations.

## SOFMMOO Recommendations

1. Prior episodes of dizziness, headache, vertigo or nausea following CSM are an absolute contraindication to further manipulation, as these symptoms indicate a high possibility of a previous dissection with a spontaneous resolution.

2. Thrust manipulations should be avoided for acute head or neck pain that is less than 3–4 days old, as this may be caused by a spontaneous VAD.

3. Neurological examination should be done on a mandatory basis as part of the pre-manipulative tests before performing any cervical thrust manipulations.

4. Rotational thrust CSM should not be performed in women under 50 years of age. In men below the age of 50, rotational thrust CSM should be avoided during the first visit; however, it may be allowed in the subsequent visit if the patient's condition is not improved. Use of mobilisations, MET (muscle energy techniques), soft-tissue cervical techniques and upper thoracic spine thrust manipulations are highly recommended instead of rotational thrust.

# References

Campos-Herrera, C.R., Scaff, M., Yamamoto, F.I. and Conforto, A.B. (2008). Spontaneous cervical artery dissection: An update on clinical and diagnostic aspects. *Arquivos de neuro-psiquiatria, 66*(4), 922–927.

Debette, S. (2014). Pathophysiology and risk factors of cervical artery dissection: What have we learnt from large hospital-based cohorts? *Current Opinion in Neurology, 27*(1), 20–28.

Fukuhara, K., Ogata, T., Ouma, S., Tsugawa, J., Matsumoto, J. *et al.* (2015). Impact of initial symptom for accurate diagnosis of vertebral artery dissection. *International Journal of Stroke, 10*(A100), 30–33.

Haldeman, S., Carey, P., Townsend, M. and Papadopoulos, C. (2002). Clinical perceptions of the risk of vertebral artery dissection after cervical manipulation: The effect of referral bias. *The Spine Journal, 2*(5), 334–342.

Haynes, M.J., Vincent, K., Fischhoff, C., Bremner, A.P., Lanlo, O. and Hankey, G.J. (2012). Assessing the risk of stroke from neck manipulation: A systematic review. *International Journal of Clinical Practice, 66*(10), 940–947.

Kim, Y.K. and Schulman, S. (2009). Cervical artery dissection: Pathology, epidemiology and management. *Thrombosis Research, 123*(6), 810–821.

Nadgir, R.N., Loevner, L.A., Ahmed, T., Moonis, G. *et al.* (2003). Simultaneous bilateral internal carotid and vertebral artery dissection following chiropractic manipulation: Case report and review of the literature. *Neuroradiology, 45*(5), 311–314.

Park, K.W., Park, J.S., Hwang, S.C., Im, S.B., Shin, W.H. and Kim, B.T. (2008). Vertebral artery dissection: Natural history, clinical features and therapeutic considerations. *Journal of Korean Neurosurgical Society, 44*(3), 109–115.

Vautravers, P.H. and Maigne, J.Y. (1999). Cervical spine manipulation and the precautionary principle. *Joint, Bone, Spine: Revue du Rhumatisme, 67*(4), 272–276.

World Health Organization (2005). *WHO Guidelines on Basic Training and Safety in Chiropractic.* Geneva: World Health Organization.

# CHAPTER 8

# Importance of Breathing in Manual Therapy

## Introduction

Breathing is the single most important function in the human body. It is one of the central aspects of our whole being. On average, we breathe 20,000 times a day (Priban, 1963). In addition, there is a positive correlation between adequate breathing and good health. Our breathing patterns reflect whether all the systems of our body, including the biomechanical, respiratory and nervous systems, are functioning properly or not (CliftonSmith and Rowley, 2011).

In manual therapy, the breathing cycle of the patient is as important as the force or pressure being employed by the practitioner. Because breathing patterns advocate relaxation responses and improve cognitive states, practitioners of manipulative therapies usually coordinate various techniques with the patient's breathing, and hence they often ask their patients to take a deep breath in and exhale while applying the techniques. However, although practitioners place a great emphasis on patient's respiration, the importance of breathing while performing a technique is rarely described in the textbooks and literature of manual therapy.

Therefore, this chapter aims to provide an insight into the importance of breathing while performing manipulative techniques. In addition, this chapter also describes the physiology of breathing, particularly what happens when we inhale and exhale, and the physiological effects of breath-holding.

# The Physiology of Breathing

In physiology, breathing is the process of absorbing oxygen ($O_2$) into our bloodstream and excreting carbon dioxide ($CO_2$) to the atmosphere. Because this process involves the exchanging of gases, it is also known as gas exchange. On an average, we take 12–20 breaths per minute (Barrett, Barman and Boitano, 2010). However, although this whole process may appear to be a simple one, it is actually much more complex.

### The Mechanism of Breathing

The mechanism of breathing is complex. Although we can temporarily suppress our breathing, we do not have complete control over it. The respiratory centres located in the pons and medulla oblongata mainly control a person's breathing rate. These centres send signals to the lungs telling them when to initiate a breath. This control is automatic, spontaneous and involuntary (Shier, Butler and Lewis, 2001).

Breathing mainly involves two phases: inhalation and exhalation.

- **Inhalation**, also called inspiration, is the process of breathing in oxygen into our lungs. During normal inhalation, the diaphragm, a domed sheet of skeletal muscle that separates the chest from the abdomen, contracts and moves downwards. The diaphragm descends towards the abdominal cavity, ultimately increasing the volume of the chest cavity. The external intercostal muscles also contract during inhalation; as a result, the ribs and sternum move upwards and outwards, expanding the rib cage. This expansion further increases chest volume. The air pressure in the lungs therefore lowers compared with the atmosphere. Since air naturally moves from areas of high pressure to low pressure, this decrease in air pressure eventually draws air into the alveoli of the lungs (Shier *et al.*, 2001; Novotny and Kravitz, 2007).

- **Exhalation**, also called expiration, is the process of breathing out carbon dioxide to the atmosphere. During exhalation, the diaphragm relaxes, and it returns to its curved position, normalising the volume of the chest cavity to its original form. On the other hand, the external intercostal muscles also relax, moving the rib and sternum downwards and inwards. As a result, the rib cage contracts, causing the chest volume to diminish. The air pressure in the lungs is therefore greater than the atmospheric pressure. This increase in pressure ultimately forces air out of the alveoli into the atmosphere (Barrett *et al.*, 2010; Standring, 2008; Novotny and Kravitz, 2007).

### Physiological Effects of Breath-Holding

The physiological effects of breath-holding on our bodies are complex. Breath-holding is a voluntary act and is influenced by many factors, including psychological state, lung stretch and respiratory chemoreflexes. If we try to hold our breath for a prolonged period of time, this could lead to lightheadedness, dizziness and unconsciousness. However, breath-holding to unconsciousness is rare, and scientific reports on this have been inconsistent (Skow *et al.*, 2015).

In general, when we voluntarily hold our breath, the arterial pressure of $O_2$ drops below its normal level, but the arterial pressure of $CO_2$ begins to rise above its usual level (Lin *et al.*, 1974). These changes in $O_2$ and $CO_2$ levels stimulate both peripheral and central chemoreceptors. The chemoreceptors then send this message to the respiratory centres in the pons and medulla, causing a respiratory drive to breathe. When this occurs, involuntary respiratory movements might also take place. However, it is not yet clear how the respiratory musculature is affected when we hold our breath. Thus, the exact changes in the diaphragm and external intercostal muscles during breath-holding have not been firmly established (Parkes, 2006).

## Importance of Breathing

Breathing is vital for our survival, as it provides our bodies with necessary oxygen and excretes waste products and toxins. Without adequate oxygen, all our organ systems would rapidly fail: the brain would stop working and blood flow would be much faster. On the other hand, if waste products are not exhaled, they could create a harsh environment in our body and damage vital functions of the cells, tissues and organs.

Thus, through breathing, we actually balance the exchanging of gases in the most efficient way (Fried, 1993).

Breathing has a positive correlation with our mind. If our breathing is normal, the mind will be calm and relaxed; however, the opposite will happen if our way of breathing is brief and irregular. Breathing is also essential to our movement and stability. The diaphragm works in unison with a number of muscles, including the internal and external obliques, transversus abdominus, multifidius, the quadratus lumborum and the pelvic floor muscles, to maintain core stability and establish intra-abdominal pressure. All these structures serve to stabilise the core and permit efficient movement and respiration (CliftonSmith and Rowley, 2011).

## Why Breathing Matters in Manual Therapy

Manual therapy practitioners, including osteopaths, chiropractors and physical therapists, provide a careful attention on their patients' breathing when they apply a technique. They usually coordinate their techniques with the patient breathing out, and there are a number of good reasons behind this. These include:

- **Breathing out is easier.** Unlike breathing in and breath-holding, breathing out is comparatively a much less stressful process of respiration. It actually requires no effort from our bodies, because the elastic recoil of the lungs passively squeezes air out. Furthermore, gravity also plays a part in pulling the ribs down during exhalation.

- **Breathing out generates a sense of relaxation.** When we take a deep breath in and slowly exhale, our mind reaches a state of tranquillity and calm. This is because deep, slow breathing activates the parasympathetic nervous system, turning down all the physiological factors that could upset the brain, including blood pressure, stress hormone level, muscle tension and heart rate.

- **Breathing out provides both posture and spinal stability.** When we exhale, the diaphragm and the external intercostal muscles relax, decreasing the volume of the chest cavity. The diaphragm has been shown to play a vital role in respiration and postural stability (Hodges and Gandevia, 2000). In unison with other muscles, it also plays a major role in establishing intra-abdominal pressure, which, if increased, could stiffen the spine.

In addition, practitioners usually coordinate their posture and breathing with the patients' respiration, so that they can make the best use of the exhalation. For this reason, they often ask the patient to exhale while they themselves breathe out.

### Why Manipulation is Not Performed during Breath-Holding

Manipulation is not performed with the patient holding their breath because it causes oxygen deficiency. Oxygen is vital for proper functioning of the body. When we hold our breath, the $O_2$ level goes down and $CO_2$ level quickly rises (Lin *et al.*, 1974). As a result, a great fluctuation in blood pressure (i.e. a sharp rise followed by a sudden drop) can occur. This can ultimately cause fatigue, poor energy, lightheadedness, dizziness and faint or blackout (Skow *et al.*, 2015). Moreover, since respiratory musculature is affected during breath-holding, employing a manipulation technique at the same time may create strain against the patient's thorax and abdomen, increase intra-abdominal pressure and disrupt the posture and spinal stability.

## References

Barrett, K.E., Barman, S.M. and Boitano, S. (2010). *Ganong's Review of Medical Physiology*. New Delhi: McGraw-Hill.

CliftonSmith, T. and Rowley, J. (2011). Breathing pattern disorders and physiotherapy: Inspiration for our profession. *Physical Therapy Reviews, 16*(1), 75–86.

Fried, R. (1993). *The Psychology and Physiology of Breathing: In Behavioral Medicine, Clinical Psychology, and Psychiatry*. New York, NY: Springer Science & Business Media.

Hodges, P.W. and Gandevia, S.C. (2000). Activation of the human diaphragm during a repetitive postural task. *The Journal of Physiology, 522*(1), 165–175.

Lin, Y.C., Lally, D.A., Moore, T.O. and Hong, S.K. (1974). Physiological and conventional breath-hold breaking points. *Journal of Applied Physiology, 37*(3), 291–296.

Novotny, S. and Kravitz, L. (2007). The science of breathing. *IDEA Fitness Journal, 4*(2), 36–43.

Parkes, M.J. (2006). Breath-holding and its breakpoint. *Experimental Physiology, 91*(1), 1–15.

Priban, I.P. (1963). An analysis of some short-term patterns of breathing in man at rest. *The Journal of Physiology, 166*(3), 425–434.

Shier, D., Butler, J. and Lewis, R. (2001). *Human Anatomy and Physiology*. New York, NY: McGraw-Hill.

Skow, R.J., Day, T.A., Fuller, J.E., Bruce, C.D. and Steinback, C.D. (2015). The ins and outs of breath holding: Simple demonstrations of complex respiratory physiology. *Advances in Physiology Education, 39*(3), 223–231.

Standring, S. (2008). *Gray's Anatomy: The Anatomical Basis of Clinical Practice*. London: Churchill Livingstone.

# PART II

# Techniques

# CHAPTER 9

# The Cervical Spine

## Introduction

Cervical spine manipulation (CSM) has been used for years to treat a multitude of head and neck disorders, including upper back pain, neck pain and stiffness, cervical disc problems, headaches and migraine. Practitioners of this therapy consider it a safe and effective manipulative procedure because of its relatively low adverse effects (Killinger, 2004). However, multiple recent studies have reported a range of serious and at times fatal complications following CSM, and suggested that the potential health risks associated with the procedure might offset the benefits (Di Fabio, 1999; Ernst, 2007; Leon-Sanchez, Cuetter and Ferrer, 2007; Gouveia, Castanho and Ferreira, 2009; Puentedura et al., 2012).

In contrast, some authors suggested that the incidence of serious adverse events after CSM is predictable, and might be attributed to poor knowledge of body biomechanics, inappropriate skills to use the techniques and inadequate examination and judgement by the practitioner (Refshauge et al., 2002; Haneline and Triano, 2005). Taken together, it can be said that it is of critical importance for a practitioner to have proper knowledge and appropriate skill before performing a first-line cervical manipulation.

Therefore, this chapter is written to describe the various joints of the cervical spine, the range of motion in these joints and appropriate special tests to diagnose serious pathology in the region. In addition, this chapter will also describe some of the common injuries to the cervical spine and the red flags for CSM.

# Joints

The cervical spine is made up of the first seven vertebrae (C1–C7) of the spinal column, beginning just below the skull and ending just above the thoracic spine. It is divided into two functionally different segments: the superior cervical segment (O–C2) and the inferior cervical segment (C3–C7). The superior segment is highly specialised and includes the occiput (O), atlas (C1) and axis (C2). The inferior cervical segment consists of more classic vertebrae, having a body, spinous processes, laminae, pedicles and facet joints (Dodwad, Khan and An, 2014).

**Table 9.1 The joints of the cervical spine**

| Joint name | Description | Function |
|---|---|---|
| Atlanto-occipital joint (O C1) | • A synovial joint of ellipsoid variety<br>• Forms due to articulation between the atlas and the occipital condyles<br>• Made up of a pair of condyloid joints | • Responsible for 50% of total neck flexion and extension<br>• Serves to maintain and support the weight and movement of the head and neck |
| Atlantoaxial joint (C1–C2) | • A complex joint consisting of three synovial joints<br>• Forms due to articulation between the atlas and axis<br>• Made up of a pair of plain joints (lateral joints) and a pivot joint (median joint) | • Responsible for 50% of all cervical rotation<br>• Serves to maintain and support the weight and movement of the head and neck |
| Lower cervical joints (C3–C7) | • Originate from the inferior surface of the axis and end at the superior surface of the first thoracic vertebra (T1)<br>• Articulations include the uncovertebral joints, disc-vertebral body and facet joints | • Responsible for 50% of total neck flexion, extension and rotation |

Sources: White and Panjabi (1990); Johnson (1991); Standring (2008)

# Range of Motion

The cervical spine is the most mobile segment of the entire spine and supports a high degree of movement. However, movements in the cervical spine are complex, as motion in one individual joint involves not just complementary but also unequal motion between cervical levels (Van Mameren *et al.*, 1989). In general, the range of motion of the cervical spine is three-dimensional:

| | |
|---|---|
| Rotation | Up to 90° (both sides) |
| Flexion | 80° to 90° (approximately) |
| Extension | 70° (approximately) |
| Lateral flexion | 20° to 45° (approximately) |

Source: Adapted from Swartz, Floyd and Cendoma (2005)

**Table 9.2 Range of motion between different cervical joints**

| Motion unit | Range of motion |
|---|---|
| O–C1 | • 25° of flexion and extension<br>• 5° of axial rotation<br>• 7° of lateral bending |
| C1–C2 | • 15° of flexion and extension<br>• 30° of axial rotation<br>• 4° or less of lateral bending |
| C2–C3 | • 8° of flexion and extension<br>• 9° of rotation<br>• 10° of lateral bending |
| C3–C4 | • 13° of flexion and extension<br>• 12° of rotation<br>• 10° of lateral bending |
| C4–C5 | • 19° of flexion and extension<br>• 12° of rotation<br>• 10° of lateral bending |

| C5–C6 | • 17° of flexion and extension<br>• 14° of rotation<br>• 8° of lateral bending |
|---|---|
| C6–C7 | • 16° of flexion and extension<br>• 10° of rotation<br>• 7° of lateral bending |

Sources: Tubbs *et al.* (2010, 2011); Schafer and Faye (1990)

# Common Injuries

A major injury to the cervical spine is often caused by a fall or motor vehicle accident. Such injuries usually lead to a fracture in the cervical vertebra, and subsequently to pain and poor spinal functioning, depending on the severity of the injury (Torretti and Sengupta, 2007). Two of the most predominantly affected cervical levels are craniocervical junction (the junction between O and C2) and the C6–C7 segment. However, most fatal cervical injuries frequently occur at the atlantoaxial joints (Trafton, 1982).

**Table 9.3 Common injuries of the cervical joints**

| Injury | Characteristics |
|---|---|
| Atlanto-occipital dislocation | • A highly unstable craniocervical injury that is associated with significant neurological morbidity and mortality<br>• May occur due to severe extension or flexion at the atlanto-occipital level<br>• Disrupts all ligamentous and/or bony connections between O and C1 |
| Jefferson fracture | • A bony fracture of the atlas caused by a compressive downward force<br>• Causes fracture of one or both of the anterior or posterior arches<br>• May cause fracture of all four aspects of the atlas ring |
| Odontoid fracture | • A fracture that occurs at the base of the dens<br>• The displacement of the fractured segment may occur anteriorly, posteriorly or laterally |

| Injury | Characteristics |
|---|---|
| Atlantoaxial subluxation | • A disorder of the C1–C2 complex that impairs neck rotation<br>• Occurs when the transverse ligament is disrupted and a rotatory component at the superior cervical segment is absent during flexion<br>• May cause neurological injury because of cord compression between the odontoid and posterior arch of atlas |
| Hangman fracture | • An unstable fracture caused by hyperextension of C2<br>• Commonly occurs due to motor vehicle collisions and results in bilateral fractures through the C2 pedicles |

Sources: Hall *et al.* (2015); Trafton (1982); Goldberg *et al.* (2001)

## Red Flags

Red flags for CSM help practitioners to make sound clinical judgements as part of the examination process. If a red flag symptom is found in a patient, the practitioner should prioritise sound clinical reasoning and exercise utmost caution, so that the patient is not placed at risk of an undue adverse event following CSM.

**Table 9.4 Red flags for cervical spine manipulation**

| Condition | Signs and symptoms |
|---|---|
| Cervical myelopathy | • Sensory disturbances in the hand<br>• Intrinsic muscle wasting of hand<br>• Clonus<br>• Babinski sign<br>• Hoffman's reflex<br>• Unsteady gait<br>• Bladder and bowel disturbances<br>• Inverted supinator sign<br>• Hyperreflexia<br>• Multisegmental sensory changes<br>• Multisegmental weakness |
| Inflammatory or systemic disease | • Gradual onset of symptoms<br>• Family history<br>• Fatigue<br>• Temperature above 100°F<br>• Blood pressure above 160/95 mmHg<br>• Resting pulse above 100bpm<br>• Resting respiration above 25bpm |

| | |
|---|---|
| Neoplastic conditions | • Over 50 years of age<br>• Previous history of cancer<br>• Constant pain that does not subside even with rest<br>• Unexplained weight loss<br>• Night pain |
| Upper cervical ligamentous instability | • Post trauma<br>• Occipital numbness and headache<br>• Severe limitation during the neck's active range of motion (AROM) in every direction<br>• Down syndrome |
| Other serious cervical pathology | • Previous diagnosis of vertebrobasilar insufficiency<br>• Dizziness/vertigo<br>• Drop attacks<br>• Ataxia<br>• Nausea<br>• Dysphasia<br>• Dysarthria<br>• Diplopia |

Sources: World Health Organization (2005); Puentedura *et al.* (2012)

## Special Tests

### Table 9.5 Special tests for assessing serious pathology in the cervical spine

| Test | Procedure | Positive sign | Interpretation |
|---|---|---|---|
| Vertebral artery test | The patient is placed in either supine lying or sitting position. The examiner slowly but passively extends and/or rotates the patient's head and neck to the maximum range of motion, keeping the patient in either supine or upright position. The examiner sustains all positions for a minimum of ten seconds while observing for symptoms associated with vertebrobasilar insufficiency. | • Dizziness<br>• Nausea and vomiting<br>• Drop attacks<br>• Temporary vision or hearing loss<br>• Pins and needles<br>• Double vision<br>• Pallor and sweating<br>• Paralysis<br>• Dysarthria | ☐ Vertebral artery compression or occlusion |

| Test | Procedure | Positive sign | Interpretation |
|---|---|---|---|
| Sharp–Purser test | With the patient seated, the examiner stands at the lateral side of the patient. The examiner places the palm of one hand on the patient's forehead, and the thumb and fingertip pads of the other hand gently hold the spinous process of the axis (C2). The patient then slowly flexes the head, performing a slight cervical nod; in unison, the examiner retracts the head in posterior direction. | • A sliding motion of the head at the posterior direction in relation to the axis<br>• A 'clunk' sound<br>• Reduction in symptoms | ☐ Atlantoaxial instability |
| Spurling's test | With the patient seated, the practitioner stands behind the patient with his hands interlocking the crown of the patient's head. The patient laterally flexes the cervical spine; at the same time, the practitioner applies a compressive force. | • Reproduction of symptoms radiating down the patient's arm | ☐ Foraminal encroachment |
| Distraction test | The patient lies supine with the head relaxed on a pillow. The examiner gently holds the axis around its neural arch with one hand and grips the occiput with the other hand. The examiner then applies gentle distraction to the head. If symptom-free in neutral plane, the test should be repeated in slight flexion and then in extension. | • Excessive vertical translation when manual traction is applied<br>• Reproduction of symptoms such as nystagmus | ☐ Tectorial membrane instability<br>☐ Upper cervical ligamentous instability |

Sources: Grant (1996); Mintken, Metrick and Flynn (2008); Hartley (1995); Osmotherly, Rivett and Rowe (2012)

# References

Di Fabio, R.P. (1999). Manipulation of the cervical spine: Risks and benefits. *Physical Therapy, 79*(1), 50–65.

Dodwad, S.N.M., Khan, S.N. and An, H.S. (2014). Cervical spine anatomy. In F.H. Shen, D. Samartzis and R.G. Fessler (Eds), *Textbook of the Cervical Spine.* Maryland Heights, MO: Elsevier Saunders.

Ernst, E. (2007). Adverse effects of spinal manipulation: A systematic review. *Journal of the Royal Society of Medicine, 100*(7), 330–338.

Goldberg, W., Mueller, C., Panacek, E., Tigges, S., Hoffman, J.R., Mower, W.R. and NEXUS Group. (2001). Distribution and patterns of blunt traumatic cervical spine injury. *Annals of Emergency Medicine, 38*(1), 17–21.

Gouveia, L.O., Castanho, P. and Ferreira, J.J. (2009). Safety of chiropractic interventions: A systematic review. *Spine, 34*(11), E405–E413.

Grant, R. (1996). Vertebral artery testing: The Australian Physiotherapy Association Protocol after 6 years. *Manual Therapy, 1*(3), 149–153.

Hall, G.C., Kinsman, M.J., Nazar, R.G., Hruska, R.T. *et al.* (2015). Atlanto-occipital dislocation. *World Journal of Orthopedics, 6*(2), p.236.

Haneline, M. and Triano, J. (2005). Cervical artery dissection. A comparison of highly dynamic mechanisms: Manipulation versus motor vehicle collision. *Journal of Manipulative and Physiological Therapeutics, 28*(1), 57–63.

Hartley, A. (1995). *Practical Joint Assessment: Upper Quadrant: A Sports Medicine Manual.* Mosby-Year Book.

Johnson, R. (1991). Anatomy of the cervical spine and its related structures. In J.S. Torg (Ed.), *Athletic Injuries to the Head, Neck, and Face.* Mosby Inc.

Killinger, L.Z. (2004). Chiropractic and geriatrics: A review of the training, role, and scope of chiropractic in caring for aging patients. *Clinics in Geriatric Medicine, 20*(2), 223–235.

Leon-Sanchez, A., Cuetter, A. and Ferrer, G. (2007). Cervical spine manipulation: An alternative medical procedure with potentially fatal complications. *Southern Medical Journal, 100*(2), 201–204.

Mintken, P.E., Metrick, L. and Flynn, T. (2008). Upper cervical ligament testing in a patient with os odontoideum presenting with headaches. *Journal of Orthopaedic and Sports Physical Therapy, 38*(8), 465–475.

Osmotherly, P.G., Rivett, D.A. and Rowe, L.J. (2012). The anterior shear and distraction tests for craniocervical instability: An evaluation using magnetic resonance imaging. *Manual Therapy, 17*(5), 416–421.

Puentedura, E.J., March, J., Anders, J., Perez, A. *et al.* (2012). Safety of cervical spine manipulation: Are adverse events preventable and are manipulations being performed appropriately? A review of 134 case reports. *Journal of Manual and Manipulative Therapy, 20*(2), 66–74.

Refshauge, K.M., Parry, S., Shirley, D., Larsen, D., Rivett, D.A. and Boland, R. (2002). Professional responsibility in relation to cervical spine manipulation. *Australian Journal of Physiotherapy, 48*(3), 171–179.

Schafer, R.C. and Faye, L.J. (1990). The cervical spine. In: *Motion palpation and chiropractic technique: Principles of Dynamic Chiropractic*. Huntington Beach, CA, Motion Palpation Institute.

Standring, S. (2008). *Gray's Anatomy: The Anatomical Basis of Clinical Practice*. London: Churchill Livingstone.

Swartz, E.E., Floyd, R.T. and Cendoma, M. (2005). Cervical spine functional anatomy and the biomechanics of injury due to compressive loading. *Journal of Athletic Training, 40*(3), 155.

Torretti, J.A. and Sengupta, D.K. (2007). Cervical spine trauma. *Indian Journal of Orthopaedics, 41*(4), 255.

Trafton, P.G. (1982). Spinal cord injuries. *The Surgical Clinics of North America, 62*(1), 61.

Tubbs, R.S., Dixon, J., Loukas, M., Shoja, M.M. and Cohen-Gadol, A.A. (2010). Ligament of Barkow of the craniocervical junction: Its anatomy and potential clinical and functional significance: Laboratory investigation. *Journal of Neurosurgery: Spine, 12*(6), 619–622.

Tubbs, R.S., Hallock, J.D., Radcliff, V., Naftel, R.P. *et al.* (2011). Ligaments of the craniocervical junction: A review. *Journal of Neurosurgery: Spine, 14*(6), 697–709.

Van Mameren, H., Drukker, J., Sanches, H. and Beursgens, J. (1989). Cervical spine motion in the sagittal plane (I) range of motion of actually performed movements, an X-ray cinematographic study. *European Journal of Morphology, 28*(1), 47–68.

White, A.A. and Panjabi, M.M. (1990). Kinematics of the spine. In: *Clinical Biomechanics of the Spine*. Philadelphia, PA: Lippincott, Williams & Wilkins.

World Health Organization (2005). *WHO Guidelines on Basic Training and Safety in Chiropractic*. Geneva: World Health Organization.

# Techniques for the Cervical Spine

## Supine Occipital Atlantal and Atlantal Axial (C0–C1/2)

- Ask the patient to lie supine with a pillow under the head.
- Stand at the head of the table.
- Fully rotate the head and then bring it back halfway to 50% of rotation.
- With your contact hand, locate the base of the ipsilateral occiput, atlas or TVP of C2.
- Your support hand should gently cradle the contralateral occipital area.
- Using the index finger MCP joint of your contact hand, apply a light contact to the desired area.
- Your other hand makes contact over the zygomatic arch.
- Maintaining a light contact, gently flex the patient's neck to tuck the chin.
- Keeping the weight of the patient's head on the pillow, begin to side-bend the patient's head over your point of contact while combining this with contralateral rotation.
- To help with this movement, you should shift your body towards the side of contact, keeping relaxed, bent knees in a lunge movement.
- Keeping your elbow tucked, ensure your arm is positioned in the direction to the line of drive.
- Engage the barrier.
- Ask the patient to inhale and exhale.

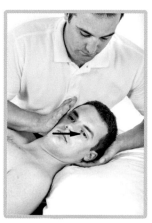

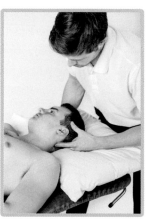

- The line of drive should be directly through the opposite occiput into side-bending with moderate traction from the support hand.
- For C1/C2, the line of drive can be slightly more rotary and directed slightly lower to affect the desired segment.

**Key Points**
- During this technique you are affecting the contralateral occiput. For a left occiput manipulation, you would contact the right occipital area and support with traction on the ipsilateral side.
- For a C1/C2, you can bias rotation of lateral flexion with your line of drive creating either increased ipsilateral lateral flexion or increased contralateral rotation.
- Light contact is key here; do not grip the patient's head or neck.
- Use distraction cues such as 'wiggle your toes' to promote full neck relaxation.
- Do not administer a manipulation until the patient has fully relaxed all muscle tension throughout the cervical spine.
- Tension should be found lightly; creating excessive tension or using excessive force through the contact or support hand will cause reflex muscle engagement.
- Use the pillow to help guide head movement; there is no need to take the full weight of the patient's head in your hands.

## C2–C7

- Ask the patient to lie supine with a pillow under the head.
- Stand at the head of the table.
- With your contact hand, locate the articular pillar of the involved spinal segment using the spinous processes to guide your anatomy.
- Your support hand should gently cradle the contralateral occipital area with the palmar aspect while supporting the contralateral aspect of the chosen spinal segment with the 1st MCP.
- Using the index finger MCP joint of your contact hand, apply a light contact to the desired area.
- Keeping the weight of the patient's head on the pillow, begin to side-bend the patient's head over your point of contact while combining this with contralateral rotation.

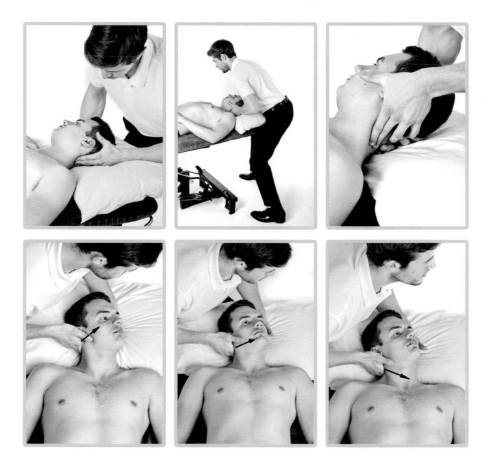

- To help with this movement, you should shift your body towards the side of contact, keeping relaxed, bent knees in a lunge movement.
- Keeping your elbow tucked, ensure your arm is positioned in the direction to the line of drive.
- Engage the barrier where the soft-tissue play has been removed and the pivot point is directly over your contact hand. This will be lower and more pronounced as you descend further through the cervical spinal segments.
- Ask the patient to inhale and exhale.
- For all cervical spine segments, the line of drive can emphasise a rotational or side-bending component and is directed lower as the spinal segments descend.
- Apply a manipulation through the contact hand, making sure the patient's head remains in slight flexion or chin tucked.

- The direction of the manipulation is dependent on the level of the cervical spine, as can be seen in the pictures.

**Key Points**

- For all cervical spine segments, you can bias rotation of side-bending with your line of drive creating either increased ipsilateral side-bending or increased contralateral rotation.
- Light contact is key here; do not grip the patient's head or neck.
- Use distraction cues such as 'wiggle your toes' to promote full neck relaxation; it may help if they do not move too much.
- Do not administer the manipulation until the patient has fully relaxed all muscle tension throughout the cervical spine.
- The barrier should be found lightly; creating excessive tension or using excessive force through the contact or support hand will cause reflex muscle engagement.
- Use the pillow to help guide head movement; there is no need to take the full weight of the patient's head in your hands at any point during the manipulation.

## Supine Recumbent C2–C7

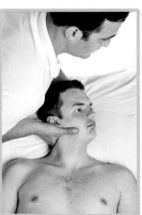

- Ask the patient to lie supine with a pillow under the head. Raise the table to around 30 degrees.
- Stand at the side of the table, ipsilateral to the side of contact.
- With your contact hand, locate the articular pillar of the involved spinal segment using the spinous processes to guide your anatomy.
- Your support hand should gently cradle the contralateral occipital area with the palmar aspect while supporting the contralateral aspect of the chosen spinal segment with the index finger.
- Using the index finger MCP joint of your contact hand, apply a light contact to the desired area.
- Take skin slack by moving your index finger medial to lateral from the spinous process.

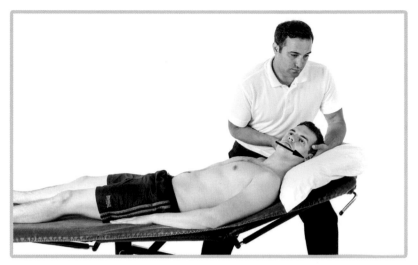

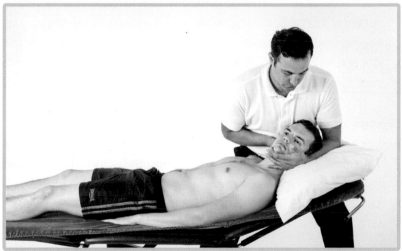

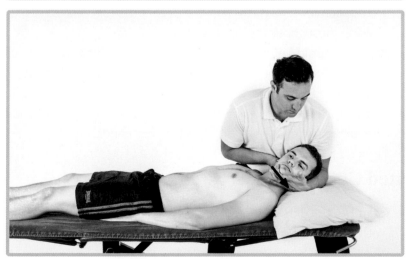

- Maintaining a light contact, gently flex the patient's neck to tuck the chin.
- Keeping the weight of the patient's head on the pillow, begin to laterally flex the patient's head over your point of contact while combining this with contralateral rotation.
- Keeping your elbow tucked, ensure your arm is positioned in the direction to the line of drive.
- Achieve a point of tension where the soft-tissue play has been removed and the pivot point is directly over your contact hand. This will be lower and more pronounced as you descend further through the cervical spinal segments.
- Ask the patient to breathe in deeply, then out.
- For all cervical spine segments, the line of drive can emphasise a rotary or lateral flexion component and is directed lower as the spinal segments descend.
- Apply a high-velocity, low-amplitude force through the contact hand, making sure the patient's head remains in slight flexion or chin tucked.

**Key Points**
- For all cervical spine segments, you can bias rotation of lateral flexion with your line of drive creating either increased ipsilateral lateral flexion or increased contralateral rotation.
- Light contact is key here; do not grip the patient's head or neck.
- Use distraction cues such as 'wiggle your toes' to promote full neck relaxation.
- Do not administer a thrust until the patient has fully relaxed all muscle tension throughout the cervical spine.
- Tension should be found lightly; creating excessive tension or using excessive force through the contact or support hand will cause reflex muscle engagement.
- Use the pillow to help guide head movement; there is no need to take the full weight of the patient's head in your hands.

## Seated Cervical Spine

- Stand to the side of the patient to which you will rotate their head, with the patient sitting comfortably.

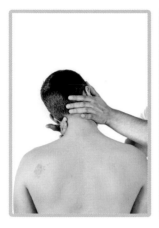 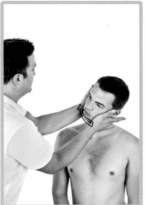 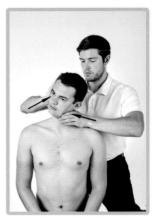

- With your contact hand, locate the chosen segment articular pillar, counting down from C2 SP.
- Finish with your 2nd and 3rd finger at the desired spinal segment to manipulate.
- Apply the support hand under the occipital area.
- Ask the patient to relax their head into your contact hand into flexion and side-bending.
- Using the contact hand, side-bend towards the contact and rotate away in a combined movement maintaining neck flexion.
- Optimise this movement, keeping your elbows in close to your body.
- Engage the barrier where the pivot point is directly over your contact.
- Ask the patient to inhale and exhale.
- Apply the manipulation at the end of exhalation.

## Alternative Contact
- Standing behind the patient, contact the involved articular pillar with the palmar aspect of your thumb. Fingers should rest lightly on the ipsilateral mandible.
- Laterally flex the patient's neck over the side of contact, including combined rotation using a similar occipital support contact.
- The elbow and forearm should be directly in line with the line of drive.

## Key Points
- Light contact is key here; do not grip the patient's head or neck.
- Use distraction cues such as 'drop your head into my hand' to promote full neck relaxation.

- Do not administer a thrust until the patient has fully relaxed all muscle tension throughout the cervical spine.
- Tension should be found lightly; creating excessive tension or using excessive force through the contact or support hand will cause reflex muscle engagement.
- Use the body and tucked elbows to help guide head movement.

## Cervico-Thoracic Junction – Side-Lying

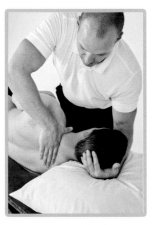

- Technique applicable to C7–T1.
- Stand in an asymmetrical stance (outside leg facing forwards), facing the patient.
- Cradle the patient's head with your forearm and your fingers resting gently over the occipital region.
- Place your other hand so that the web of your hand contacts the base of the patient's neck and the 1st MCP joint of your thumb is contacting the TP of T1.
- Ask your patient to inhale and then slowly exhale.
- As the patient exhales, begin to take up the slack in the tissues by gently raising the patient's head from the pillow, while simultaneously bending your back knee to introduce a counter pressure through your 1st MCP contact on the TP.

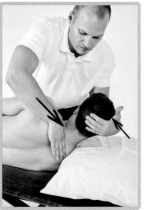

- Feel for forces localising at the target segment (engagement of barrier).
- A manipulation is delivered through the TP towards the head of the couch; at the same time introduce an equal counter force with the arm cradling the head.

### Key Points
- With the cradling arm, small amounts of cervical extension, flexion or rotation may be required to engage the barrier.

- You may want to contact the patient's forehead to aid stability.
- Use of an asymmetrical stance and bending through the back knee allows the practitioner greater control of the pressure exerted on the TP when delivering the thrust.

## Cervico-Thoracic Junction – Prone – Specific Contact with Thumb against SP

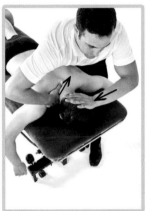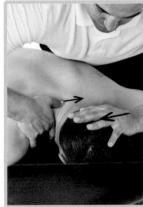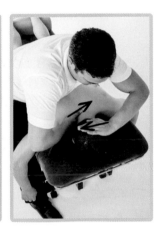

- This technique is described as shown.
- The patient is in the prone position with arms over the side of the table.
- The practitioner stands in a split-leg stance with the left leg in front.
- Locate the SP of T1.
- With your right hand, rest the web of your hand over the patient's trapezius and gently but firmly place the pad of your thumb against the side of the target SP.
- Place your left hand against the side of the patient's head just above the ear, ensuring your forearm is as near to parallel with the head of the couch as possible.
- Ask the patient to inhale and then slowly exhale.
- As the patient starts to exhale, begin to introduce a side-bending force with your right hand through T1 as your left hand simultaneously introduces a rotational force to engage the barrier.
- When the barrier has been engaged, a manipulation is applied through both hands.

135

**Key Points**

- Note that this technique can be carried out from either side of the table depending on practitioner preference.
- Supporting the patient's arms with towels to avoid compression on the bicep aids their comfort.
- You may wish to use your lead leg to slightly abduct the patient's arm in order to relax the patient's trapezius.
- When applying this manipulation, you must make sure you are applying an equal and opposite force against the side of the SP.

## Cervico-Thoracic Junction – Prone – Broad Contact over Superior Angle of Scapular

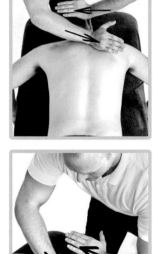

- The patient is asked to lie in the prone position.
- Ensure you have an asymmetrical stance with your lead leg in contact with the couch.
- Place the web of your hand firmly but gently against the superior angle of the contralateral scapula. Your hand should be relaxed.
- With your other hand, make contact with patient's head at the mastoid process and temporal bone.
- Have a slight bend in your knees and not your trunk.
- Ensure your forearm on the superior angle of the scapula is in line with the direction of thrust, while the other fore-arm is as near to parallel with the head of the table as possible.
- Ask the patient to inhale and then slowly exhale.
- As the patient begins to exhale, begin to take up the slack in the tissues by slowly introducing an oblique force through the patient's scapular

towards their axilla, while your other hand simultaneously introduces a rotational force parallel to the head of the couch.

- When the forces are localised to the target segment (the barrier engaged), a manipulation is applied through the rotation of the cervical spine while maintaining an equal pressure against the superior angle of the scapula.

**Key Points**

- The lead leg is generally matching the hand in contact with the superior angle of the scapula.
- To localise the forces at the target segment, use an equal pressure through both hands.
- Ensure there is equal pressure through the superior angle of the scapular so the tissues do not come off slack and engagement of the barrier lost.
- Note that a more localised applicator can be made by using the pisiform.

# Cervico-Thoracic Junction – Ipsilateral Contact

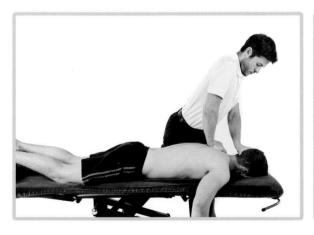
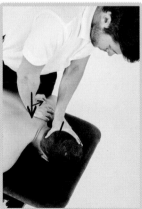

- This technique is described as shown in the pictures.
- With the patient lying prone, stand with an asymmetrical stance (left leg forward) at the ipsilateral side of the couch.

- Place the pisiform of the right hand firmly but gently on the TP of the target segment (T1).
- Ensure your elbow is locked and your bodyweight is directly over the top of TP.
- Your left hand should contact the patient's head just behind the ear, covering the temporal bone and possibly mastoid process.
- Ask the patient to inhale and then slowly exhale.
- As the patient begins to exhale, begin to take up the slack in the tissues by applying a posterior-anterior (PA) force through the pisiform while simultaneously creating a rotational movement at the TP by internally rotating the arm at the glenohumeral joint.
- The left hand should be introducing a simultaneous ipsilateral rotation of the cervical spine.
- As the forces localise to the target segment, a rotational manipulation is delivered through the left hand while the right hand simultaneously applies a combined PA and rotational movement to the TP.

**Key Points**
- Delivery of the manipulation must be done simultaneously and with the same amount of force through both hands.
- Reverse the technique for the other side.

## Cervico-Thoracic Junction – Seated

- This technique is described as shown in the photographs.
- Stand behind the seated patient.
- Adjust the height of the couch so that your leg can comfortably support the patient's upper right arm at 90 degrees of abduction in order to relax the patient's upper trapezius.
- Place the thumb of your left hand on the lateral side of the SP of T1.
- The fingers of the left hand should be slightly spread, with the fingertips resting comfortably on the patient's clavicle.
- Place the palm of your right hand on the temporal surface of the patient's head just above the ear.
- Ask the patient to inhale and then slowly exhale.

- Begin to take up the slack in the tissues by slowly introducing cervical side-bending by gently applying a lateral to medial force to the side of the TP, while allowing the patient's body weight to move to the right.
- As side-bending is introduced, an equal counter force is applied through the flat of the right hand.
- As the forces localise to the target segment, the manipulation is delivered through the TP in the direction of the patient's opposite axilla.

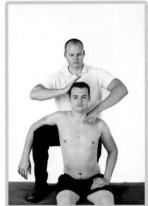

**Key Points**

- You may place a pillow under the patient's abducted arm for comfort.
- As cervical side-bending is introduced, keep the head centred with the sacrum.
- Small amounts of cervical extension, flexion or rotation maybe required to engage the barrier.

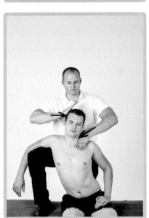

- Ensure when delivering the thrust through the TP that the other hand delivers a counter force so that the engagement of the barrier is not lost.

## Cervico-Thoracic Junction – Seated Lift Technique

- Ask the patient to sit in the middle of the couch and as far towards you as possible.
- Ask the patient to place their hands behind their neck with their fingers interlaced.
- Standing behind the patient, place a small folded or rolled towel between your sternum/chest and the vertebra below the target segment.

- Using an asymmetrical stance (which leg is forward depends on personal preference), place both arms under the patient's axillae, gently holding the patient's wrists or covering their fingers with yours interlaced.
- Ask the patient to inhale and then slowly exhale.
- As the patient begins to exhale, gently lean the patient back towards you by transferring your weight onto your back leg.
- Feel for a gradual increase in pressure between your sternum/chest and the target segment.
- Ask the patient to look up slightly (this to avoid any additional force through the cervical spine). As the patient looks up, draw both shoulders towards you to avoid excessive movement in the shoulder and to help focus the manipulation to the target area. At the same time ask the patient to attempt to bring their elbows to the midline with 25% (approximately) of their strength. This helps as the trapezius contracts and aids in making the technique more specific.
- As the forces localise to the target segment, rapidly transfer your weight on to the lead leg by pushing up on to the ball of your back foot, as you simultaneously lift your chest in a superior PA direction to manipulate.

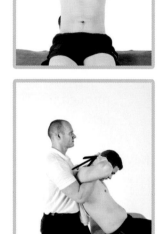

**Key Points**
- To be successful, the thrust must be made using the legs and chest/sternum and not by the practitioner trying to lift the patient upwards via their axillae.

- The technique is called a 'lift' because it lifts the superior vertebral segment off the vertebra below, not because you need to lift the patient skywards.
- If using a towel, be careful that it is not too thick as this will absorb your thrusting force and prevent the success of the manipulation.
- Practice of this technique is essential to master the multiple facets and explanation.
- Always do a run through with the patient to show them what you need them to do; the technique will be much easier for you if the patient knows what they are doing and what to expect.

# CHAPTER 10

# The Thoracic Spine

## Introduction

Thoracic spine manipulation (TSM) mainly involves high-velocity, low-amplitude (HVLA) thrust techniques being applied at any segment of the thoracic region. The therapy has been practised for years by different professions to treat a number of musculoskeletal conditions, including non-specific neck disorders, subacromial pain syndrome, kyphosis, scoliosis and juvenile kyphosis (Ombregt, 2013).

Although clinical pain syndromes in the thoracic region are less common compared with the cervical and lumbar regions, regionally interdependent musculoskeletal disorders are very common in the thoracic spine (e.g. upper thoracic immobility is often associated with neck conditions) (Walser, Meserve and Boucher, 2013). However, it is not yet fully understood why regional interdependence exists between different segments of the spine (Wainner *et al.*, 2007). Moreover, there is limited evidence in support of TSM in regions adjacent to the thoracic spine. Given the lack of high-quality literature, the benefits and risks associated with TSM are not yet fully explored (Lemole *et al.*, 2002).

This chapter is written to describe common injuries to the thoracic spine, the red flags for serious pathology and appropriate special tests to diagnose serious pathology in the region. In addition, this chapter will also describe various thoracic joints and their range of motion.

# Joints

The thoracic spine is located in the middle segment of the spinal column, between the cervical spine in the neck and the lumbar spine in the lower back. It is made up of twelve vertebrae (T1–T12), which caudally increase in size, reflecting the caudal increase in body load (McKenzie and May, 2006). These vertebrae are generally intermediate in size compared with vertebrae of other segments of the spine. The size and shape of the upper thoracic vertebrae closely resembles the cervical vertebrae. Conversely, the lower thoracic vertebrae are more similar to the lumbar vertebrae (White and Panjabi, 1978).

**Table 10.1 The joints of the thoracic spine**

| Joint name | Description | Function |
|---|---|---|
| Costovertebral joint | • A synovial joint that connects the head of the rib with the costal facets of adjacent vertebral bodies and the intervertebral disc in between<br>• Composed of a fibrous capsule, the fan-shaped radiate ligament and the interarticular ligament | • Serves to support spinal movement<br>• Helps the ribs to work in a parallel fashion while breathing |
| Costotransverse joint | • Forms when the tubercle of the rib articulates with the transverse process of the corresponding vertebra<br>• Consists of a capsule, the neck and tubercle ligaments, and the costotransverse ligaments<br>• Absent in T11 and T12 | • Helps the ribs to work in a parallel fashion while breathing |
| Zygapophyseal joints | • A set of synovial joints that are formed by joining the articular processes of two neighbouring vertebrae | • Serve to restrain the amount of flexion and anterior translation of the vertebral segment<br>• Guide and constrain the motion of the vertebrae<br>• Facilitate rotation |

Sources: Duprey *et al.* (2010); Pal, Routal and Saggu (2001); Bontrager and Lampignano (2013)

## Range of Motion

The thoracic spine is the least mobile segment of the vertebral column, because of its articulations with the rib cage. Moreover, it is technically difficult to measure thoracic movements. For this reason, unlike its other spinal counterparts, studies done to evaluate the movement of the thoracic spine are very limited.

**Table 10.2 Range of motion in the thoracic spine**

| Movement type | Motion unit | Range of motion |
| --- | --- | --- |
| Flexion | C7–T1 | 9° (approximately) |
| | T1–T6 | 4° |
| | T6–T7 | 4–8° |
| | T12–L1 | 8–12° |
| Lateral bending | T1–T10 | 6° (approximately) |
| | T11–L1 | 8° (approximately) |
| Sagittal | T1–T10 | Less than 5° |
| | T10–T12 | 5° (approximately) |
| Rotation | T1–T4 | 8–12° |
| | T5–T8 | 8° (approximately) |
| | T9–T12 | Less than 3° |

Sources: McKenzie and May (2006); Leahy and Rahm (2007)

## Common Injuries

Injuries to the thoracic spine usually occur when external forces applied on the vertebral column go beyond its strength and stability. Common causes of injuries include a fall, motor vehicle accident, violent activity, sport accident and penetrating trauma. Such injuries usually lead to a fracture in the thoracic vertebrae, and subsequently to pain and poor spinal functioning, depending on the severity of the injury.

**Table 10.3 Common injuries of the thoracic joints**

| Injury | Characteristics |
|---|---|
| Compression fracture | • Causes the anterior part of the vertebra to break and lose height<br>• Usually a stable fracture, as it does not move the bones out of their places<br>• Does not cause neurologic problems<br>• Commonly occurs in osteoporosis patients |
| Vertebral body fracture | • Most common in the thoracolumbar region<br>• Often results from a high-energy accident or osteoporosis<br>• May also occur because of an underlying disorder, such as ankylosing spondylitis, a vertebral tumour or infection<br>• Symptoms include pain or the development of neural deficits such as numbness, weakness, tingling, spinal shock and neurogenic shock<br>• More predominant in men than women |
| Fracture-dislocation | • A severe injury in which a thoracic vertebra fractures and moves off an adjacent vertebra<br>• Usually an unstable injury<br>• Often causes compression of the spinal cord |
| Transverse process fracture | • Usually results from rotation or extreme lateral bending<br>• Often occurs due to a direct blow to the thoracic region<br>• Does not affect the spinal stability |

Sources: Kostuik *et al.* (1991); Ombregt (2013)

## Red Flags

Red flags help to identify serious pathology in patients with thoracic pain. If a red flag symptom is found in a patient, the practitioner should prioritise sound clinical reasoning and exercise utmost caution, so that the patient is not placed at risk of an undue adverse event following TSM.

## Table 10.4 Red flags for serious pathology in the thoracic spine

| Condition | Signs and symptoms |
|---|---|
| Spinal tumours | • Greater than 50 years of age<br>• Past history of cancer<br>• Unintentional weight loss<br>• Constant progressive pain at night<br>• Pain lasting for more than a month<br>• No improvement after a month of conventional treatment |
| Spinal infection | • Greater than 50 years of age<br>• Recent bacterial infection such as respiratory, urinary tract or skin infection, tuberculosis<br>• History of intravenous drug abuse<br>• Persistent fever or systemic illness |
| Spinal cord lesion | • Dysfunction of bowel or bladder<br>• Positive Babinski sign<br>• Motor weakness, loss of dexterity, disturbed gait, clumsiness<br>• Paraesthesia |
| Fracture | • Greater than 70 years of age<br>• Recent history of major trauma<br>• Prolonged use of corticosteroids<br>• History of osteoporosis |
| Inflammatory arthropathy | • Gradual onset: less than 40 years of age<br>• Family history<br>• Morning stiffness for longer than one hour<br>• Persisting limitation of movement<br>• Involvement of peripheral joint<br>• Iritis, colitis, skin rashes or urethral discharge |
| Vascular/ neurological | • Excessive dizziness<br>• Blackouts or falls<br>• Positive cranial nerve signs |

Sources: Nachemson and Vingard (2000); Ombregt (2003); McKenzie and May (2006)

## Special Tests

### Table 10.5 Special tests for assessing serious pathology in the thoracic spine

| Test | Procedure | Positive sign | Interpretation |
|------|-----------|---------------|----------------|
| Cervical rotation lateral flexion test | With the patient in seated position, the examiner stands behind the patient. The examiner passively and maximally rotates the head away from the affected side. The examiner then attempts to laterally flex the head as far as possible, moving the ear towards the chest. | • Inability to laterally flex the head | ☐ 1st rib hypomobility in patients with brachialgia |
| Passive rotation test | With the patient in seated position, the examiner stands in front of the patient. The examiner asks the patient to cross both arms across the chest and holds the patient's knees between his/her legs to immobilise the pelvis. The examiner then twists the patient's trunk towards the left and the right. At the end of each rotation, the examiner asks the patient to bend the head actively forwards. The examiner notes the severity of pain, range of motion and end-feel. | • A hard end-feel<br>• An empty end-feel with muscle spasm<br>• Increased pain during movement of the head | ☐ A hard end-feel is often suggestive of ankylosing spondylitis or advanced arthrosis<br>☐ An empty end-feel with muscle spasm suggest a severe disorder (e.g. neoplasm)<br>☐ Increased pain during movement of the head is regarded as a dural sign |

| Test | Procedure | Positive sign | Interpretation |
|---|---|---|---|
| Anterior-posterior rib compression test | The patient can be in either seated or standing position. The therapist stands laterally to the patient and places one hand on the anterior and another on the posterior aspects of the rib cage. The therapist compresses the rib cage by pushing the hands together and then releases the pressure. | • The rib shaft being prominent in the midaxillary line<br>• Pain or point tenderness with the rib-cage compression<br>• Respiratory restrictions for both inhalation and exhalation | ☐ Possibly a rib fracture, contusion or separation |
| Brudzinski's sign | With the patient lying in supine, the examiner places one hand behind the patient's head and the other hand on the patient's chest. The examiner then passively flexes the patient's neck by pulling head to chest, while restraining the body from rising. | • Involuntary flexion of the patient's hips and knees | ☐ Meningeal irritation |

Sources: Lindgren et al. (1990); Ombregt (2013); Magee (2002); Saberi and Syed (1999)

# References

Bontrager, K.L. and Lampignano, J. (2013). *Textbook of Radiographic Positioning and Related Anatomy*. St Louis, MO: Elsevier Health Sciences.

Duprey, S., Subit, D., Guillemot, H., and Kent, R.W. (2010). Biomechanical properties of the costovertebral joint. *Medical Engineering and Physics, 32*(2), 222–227.

Kostuik, J., Huler, R., Esses, S. and Stauffer, S. (1991). Thoracolumbar spine fracture. In *The Adult Spine: Principles and Practice*. New York, NY: Raven Press.

Leahy, M. and Rahm, M. (2007). Thoracic spine fractures and dislocations. *eMedicine*, 12.

Lemole, G.M., Bartolomei, J., Henn, J.S. and Sonntag, V.K.H. (2002). Thoracic fractures. In A.R. Vaccaro (Ed.), *Fractures of the Cervical, Thoracic, and Lumbar Spine*. Boca Raton, FL: CRC Press.

Lindgren, K.A., Leino, E., Hakola, M. and Hamberg, J. (1990). Cervical spine rotation and lateral flexion combined motion in the examination of the thoracic outlet. *Archives of Physical Medicine and Rehabilitation, 71*(5), 343–344.

Magee, D.J. (2002). *Orthopedic Physical Assessment*, 4th edition. St Louis, MO: Elsevier Health Sciences.

McKenzie, R. and May, S. (2006). *The Cervical and Thoracic Spine: Mechanical Diagnosis and Therapy*. Windham, NH: Orthopedic Physical Therapy Products.

Nachemson, A. and Vingard, E. (2000). Assessment of patients with neck and back pain: A best-evidence synthesis. In A.L. Nachemson and E. Jonsson (Eds), *Neck and Back Pain: The Scientific Evidence of Causes, Diagnosis, and Treatment*. Philadelphia, PA: Lippincott Williams & Wilkins.

Ombregt, L. (2013). *Clinical Examination of the Thoracic Spine: A System of Orthopaedic Medicine*. St Louis, MO: Elsevier Health Sciences.

Pal, G.P., Routal, R.V. and Saggu, S.K. (2001). The orientation of the articular facets of the zygapophyseal joints at the cervical and upper thoracic region. *Journal of Anatomy, 198*(04), 431–441.

Saberi, A. and Syed, S.A. (1999). Meningeal signs: Kernig's sign and Brudzinski's sign. *Hospital Physician, 35*, 23–26.

Wainner, R.S., Whitman, J.M., Cleland, J.A. and Flynn, T.W. (2007). Regional interdependence: A musculoskeletal examination model whose time has come. *Journal of Orthopaedic and Sports Physical Therapy, 37*(11), 658–660.

Walser, R.F., Meserve, B.B. and Boucher, T.R. (2013). The effectiveness of thoracic spine manipulation for the management of musculoskeletal conditions: A systematic review and meta-analysis of randomized clinical trials. *Journal of Manual and Manipulative Therapy, 17*(4), 237–246.

White, A.A. and Panjabi, M.M. (1978). *Clinical Biomechanics of the Spine*. Philadelphia, PA: J.B. Lippincott Company.

# Techniques for the Thoracic Spine

## Hand Positioning for Thoracic Manipulation

The ability to adapt your hand position is an important factor in manipulative therapy. You should be able to adapt your hand position depending on the type of manipulation you wish to perform, and to the area of the spine you are working on and for the patient you are working with.

There are four hand positions that you can use and some adaptions that can be implemented to avoid compromising your contact hand if you have larger or heavier patients.

### Flat Palm

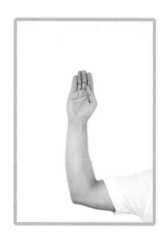

- This is a softer hand position for manipulation techniques for the patient.
- You will move your thumb between the first and second phalange, creating a small fulcrum.
- For thoracic manipulation and rib manipulation, the spinous processes (SPs) of the target segment will sit within the groove of the mid-palm.

### The Pistol

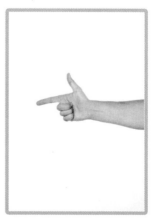

- The pistol grip is a staple hand position for thoracic and rib techniques.
- The thumb and index finger create the image of a pistol with the remaining fingers folding in to create a deep sulcus within the palm.
- The SPs of the target segments will sit in that sulcus.

- Your index finger should remain level with the transverse process (TP) of the target segment but keeping the elbow at 90 degrees.

## Closed Hand

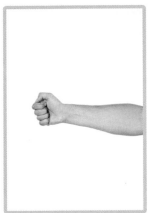

- The closed hand is a more robust hand position. You create a fist, ensuring that your thumb sits above the index finger and not on it as that could compromise your thumb during the manipulation. The closed hand allows the target SPs to sit nicely in the sulcus between the fingers and the palm.
- If you find that your hand hurts during any thoracic manipulation using the closed hand, you can hold on to a thin towel to give additional cushioning and support during the technique.

## Concealed Thumb

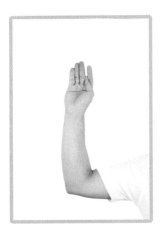

- The concealed thumb is more effective for upper rib manipulation.
- You will move your thumb and place it between the first two fingers.
- This creates a much deeper sulcus; the SPs sit within that sulcus to allow an effectively manipulation.

# Prone Thoracic Thrust – 'Butterfly'

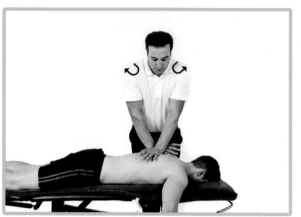
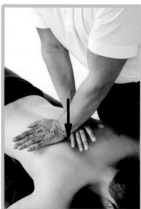

- This technique is applicable between T2 and T10.
- Ask the patient to lie in the prone position.
- The practitioner stands at the side of the table, facing the patient.
- Ensure you have an asymmetrical stance with your lead leg in contact with the table.
- Locate the target segment.
- Your dominant hand should contact the TP of the target segment on the ipsilateral side via your pisiform.
- With the other hand, contact the TP of the segment below your target on the contralateral side via your pisiform creating your 'butterfly' wings (e.g. ipsilateral contact on T3 and contralateral contact on T4).
- While adding minimal contact on the patient, ask them to inhale.
- As the patient exhales, begin to move your bodyweight over the target segment. Imagine you are aiming to place your xiphoid process over the SP.
- As you follow the exhalation phase, you add equal bilateral compression through both arms, which are at almost full extension, and external rotation of both shoulders to gather any skin slack.
- As the patient reaches full exhalation, apply your manipulation towards the table.

**Key Points**

- For patient comfort, you may want to place a small towel under each shoulder.
- Breathing is key. Allow the patient to inhale while you apply minimal compression; as they exhale, gradually increase compression by moving your body weight forward over the target segment.
- At the full end point of exhalation, ensuring there is minimal air left in the lungs, apply your manipulation.

## Supine Thoracic Manipulation T2–T12

- Technique can be applied to T2–T12 in supine.
- You need to adopt an asymmetrical stance.
- The patient crosses their arms into a V position. The opposite arm to the side you are standing on should be the lowest elbow.
- Palpate the opposite medial border of the scapula to expose the SPs of the thoracic spine.
- Using you chosen applicator, contact the segment below your target (i.e. T6 to manipulate T5).
- Your other hand now gently holds the two elbows as you will need to control this to complete the manipulation.
- The patient should now inhale and exhale.
- Halfway through the exhalation phase, roll the patient on to your applicator.
- As you roll the patient on to your applicator, you compress the elbows via your xiphoid process.
- The aim is to direct the patient's elbows directly above your applicator.
- At the end of the exhalation phase, maximum compression via the elbows should be achieved and the manipulation should be completed.
- The direction of the manipulation is SO through the shoulders.

**Key Points**

- You can assess your target segment by palpating the SPs and gently and slowly rocking the patient on and off your hand.

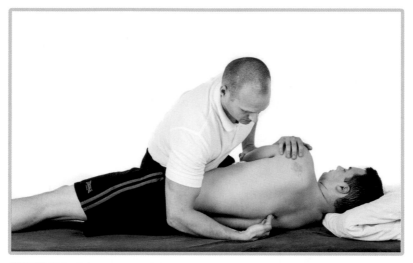

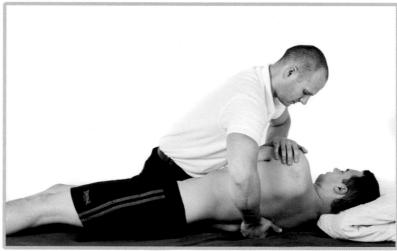

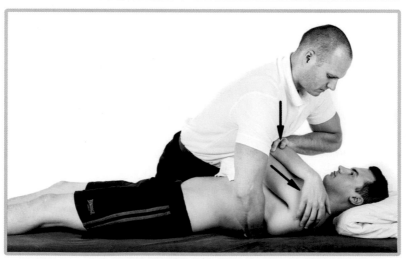

- A towel can be placed under the crossed arms for people with longer arms or very mobile shoulders.
- A towel can be placed over the patient's elbows to enable a protective cushion for the practitioner.
- The plinth height is very important, requiring enough room to manipulate.

## Prone Thoracic Spear Technique

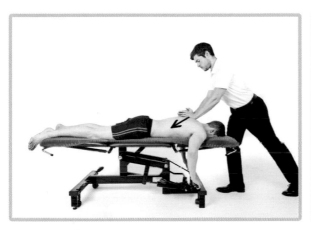

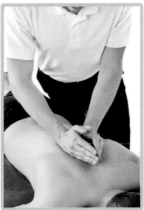

- This technique is applicable to T2–T12.
- This technique can be applied with the practitioner at either side of the table or at the head of the table.
- The technique can be applied AS or PI from the top of the table.
- You should adopt an asymmetrical stance.
- Your applicator (bilateral lateral aspect of pisiform) should contact the TP of the target with both arms at almost full extension.

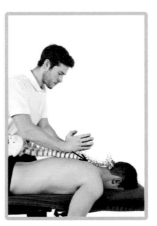

- You should aim to have your xiphoid process over the target segment as much as possible.
- Ask the patient to inhale and exhale.

- Halfway through the exhalation phase, begin to engage the barrier by adding a downward and oblique compression.
- At the end of the exhalation phase, the barrier should be engaged and you should manipulate the target joint.

**Key Points**
- Bend your knees and not your trunk in order to add the necessary compression to engage the barrier.
- Remember to work with the patient's breathing.
- Add the full downward compression at the very end of exhalation.

# Rolling Supine Thoracic Manipulation

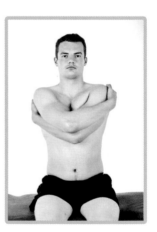

- This technique is applicable between T7 and T12.
- Raise the head of the plinth to approximately 30° to support the patient's head as they are rolled towards the table.
- The patient begins seated with one hip and knee flexed on to the table as shown.
- The patient is asked to fold their arms so their elbows meet in the centre, creating a V shape.
- A support can be used if required (towel pictured) when moving the patient towards the table to enhance the fulcrum created by your hand.
- You stand to the side of the table with an asymmetrical stance.
- You place your chosen applicator either flat palm, fist grip or pistol grip below the level you intend to manipulate (e.g. T6 to manipulate T5).
- You contact the patient's lower elbow, securing both arms against the patient's chest.
- The patient is asked to inhale and exhale.

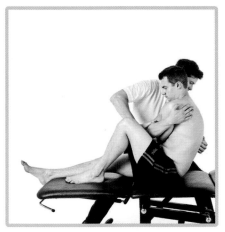 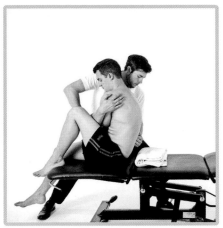

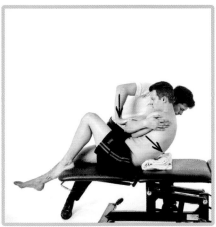 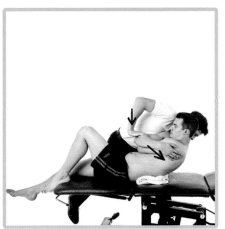

- As the patient begins to exhale, the practitioner begins lower the patient towards the table.
- When the dorsal aspect of your hand makes contact with the towel, add compression with your body through the lower elbow and manipulate the target segment.
- The manipulation is created by applying an OP force over the target segment.

**Key Points**

- Timing is everything with this technique and it will take time to master.
- The towel is used to increase your fulcrum and also to protect your hand from the table.

- You can have the patient hold a towel between their folded arms to close the gap between their chest and elbows.
- Whichever applicator you choose, the SP should lie along the palm, central to the thumb and fingers.
- The bending of the knee helps to protect the patient's lumbar spine.
- You may choose this technique if the patient is much bigger than you, as you can use momentum and gravity to help you engage the barrier.

## Seated Thoracic Lift Technique

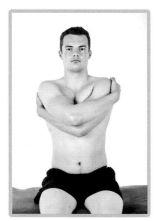
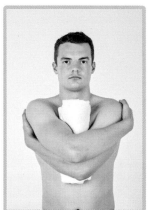
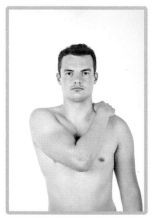
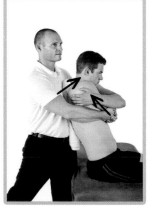

- This technique is performed seated and is applicable to T7–T12.
- You need to have an asymmetrical stance and stand behind the patient.
- The patient sits as far back on the plinth as possible, with the practitioner and patient facing away from each other.

- The patient is asked to fold as shown.
- Contact the SP of the segment below your target via a rolled-up towel.
- Place both hands over the patient's lower elbow, interlocking your fingers.
- Ask the patient to inhale and exhale.
- Towards the end of the exhalation phase, compress the patient via their elbows to remove any slack through the shoulders in a PAS direction.
- Once the barrier is engaged, perform the manipulation.

**Key Points**

- Make sure patient is not slouching prior to starting and assessing the target segment.
- The lower the target segment, the more you will be required to flex the patient from their trunk and not to put them in more lumbar extension.
- Do not perform this manipulation if there is shoulder pathology; use an alternative technique.

# CHAPTER 11

# The Lumbar Spine

## Introduction

Lumbar spine manipulation (LSM) is an intervention commonly used by practitioners of different professions (e.g. osteopathy, chiropractic and physical therapy) to treat low back pain (LBP). In patients with LBP, LSM is shown to result in rapid and prolonged reductions in spinal pain and disability (Cleland *et al.*, 2006). In addition, the therapy is considered relatively safe and effective in the treatment of individuals with LBP, because serious complications following LSM are rare. According to Oliphant (2004), the rate of serious adverse event due to LSM is 1 per 3.7 million. However, since LBP is a disorder with variable etiologies, it is of critical importance for a practitioner to diagnose the exact spinal pathology accurately before performing spinal manipulation (Majlesi *et al.*, 2008).

Therefore, this chapter is written to describe common injuries to the lumbar spine, the red flags for serious pathology and appropriate special tests to diagnose serious pathology in the region. In addition, this chapter will also describe various lumbar joints and their range of motion.

## Joints

The anatomy of the lumbar spine is complex. It is made up of five moveable vertebrae (designated L1 to L5), the intervertebral discs, large muscles, flexible ligament or tendons and highly sensitive nerves. The lumbar vertebrae are characterised by their large, thick vertebral bodies, short spinous processes and thin transverse processes. They are distinguished from their other spinal counterparts by the absence of transverse foramina and costal facets (Standring, 2008).

Functionally, the lumbar spine is designed to be incredibly strong, flexible and stable. It protects the spinal cord and spinal nerve roots by allowing a wide range of motions and serving to help support the weight of the body (Kishner, Moradian and Morello, 2014).

## Table 11.1 The joints of the lumbar spine

| Joint name | Description | Function |
|---|---|---|
| Symphyseal joints | • Also known as secondary cartilaginous joints<br>• Formed between the bodies of adjacent vertebrae of the vertebral column | • Serve to allow small movement between the adjacent vertebrae<br>• Support the body during high-impact activities or when carrying heavy objects |
| Zygapophyseal joints | • A set of synovial joints that are formed joining the superior and inferior articular processes of two neighbouring vertebrae | • Serve to restrain the amount of flexion and anterior translation of the vertebral segment<br>• Guide/allow simple gliding movements<br>• Facilitate rotation |
| Fibrous joints | • Formed when the adjacent bones of the vertebral column are directly connected to one another by fibrous connective tissue<br>• Join the laminae, transverse and spinous processes of the lumbar vertebrae | • Serve to hold the vertebral column in position |

Sources: OpenStax (2013); Standring (2008); Watson, Paxinos and Kayalioglu (2009)

# Range of Motion

In general, the movements available at the lumbar spine are principally flexion, extension, lateral flexion and axial rotation. Flexion and extension usually occur due to a combination of rotation and translation in the sagittal plane between each vertebra (Hansen *et al.*, 2006).

However, the movements at the lumbar spine are difficult to measure clinically, because they vary considerably from person to person. Moreover, a number of factors also play a part while measuring the range of motion, including age, sex, genetics, pathology and ligamentous laxity (McKenzie and May, 2003).

**Table 11.2 Range of motion in the lumbar spine**

| Motion type | Range of motion |
|---|---|
| Flexion | 40–60° |
| Extension | 20–35° |
| Lateral flexion | 15–20° |
| Rotation | 3–18° |

Source: Adapted from Magee (2014)

**Table 11.3 Segmental range of motion in males aged 25 to 36 years (based on three-dimensional radiography technique)**

| Mean range (in degrees) | | | | | | | |
|---|---|---|---|---|---|---|---|
| Interspace | Flexion | Extension | Flexion and extension | Lateral flexion | | Axial rotation | |
| | | | | Left | Right | Left | Right |
| L1–L2 | 8 | 5 | 13 | 5 | 6 | 1 | 1 |
| L2–L3 | 10 | 3 | 13 | 5 | 6 | 1 | 1 |
| L3–L4 | 12 | 1 | 13 | 5 | 6 | 1 | 2 |
| L4–L5 | 13 | 2 | 16 | 3 | 5 | 1 | 2 |
| L5–S1 | 9 | 5 | 14 | 0 | 2 | 1 | 0 |

Sources: Pearcy and Tibrewal (1984); Pearcy, Portek and Shepherd (1984)

# Common Injuries

Injuries to the lumbar spine are not rare. They usually occur when external forces applied on the vertebral column go beyond its strength and stability. Common causes of injuries include a fall, violent activity, motor vehicle accident, sport accident and penetrating trauma. Most often, lumbar spine injuries show up with a mild muscle sprain or strain. Severe injuries of the lumbar region include various types of fracture, spondylolisthesis and disc herniations (Dunn, Proctor and Day, 2006).

**Table 11.4 Common injuries of the lumbar spine**

| Injury | Characteristics |
|---|---|
| Muscle strain | • Generally refers to an injury to a muscle or tendon in the lumbar region<br>• Typical symptoms include local bruising without radiculopathy<br>• Symptoms are often exacerbated by twisting, bending and weight bearing |
| Lumbar disc herniation | • Usually occurs due to wear and tear of the disc<br>• Incidence rate is high in individuals who are exposed to substantial axial loading, rotation and flexion<br>• Symptoms include dull or sharp pain, sciatica, muscle spasm or cramping, numbness and weakness, and loss of leg function<br>• More common in athletes and older adults |
| Spondylolisthesis | • Usually occurs at L-5 (L5–S1)<br>• Often results from activities that involve repetitive hyperextension and axial loading<br>• Common symptoms include LBP without radiculopathy<br>• Symptoms may be exacerbated by extension<br>• More common in adolescents and young athletes |
| Compression fracture | • Causes the anterior part of the vertebra to break and lose height<br>• Usually a stable fracture, as it does not move the bones out of their places<br>• Does not cause neurologic problems<br>• Commonly occurs in osteoporosis patients |

| Injury | Characteristics |
|---|---|
| Vertebral body fracture | • Usually occurs due to a high-energy accident or osteoporosis<br>• Symptoms include pain or the development of neural deficits such as numbness, weakness, tingling, spinal shock and neurogenic shock<br>• More common in the thoracolumbar region<br>• More predominant in men than women |

Sources: Dunn *et al.* (2006); Ombregt (2013)

# Red Flags

Red flags help to identify serious pathology in patients with lumbar pain. If a red flag symptom is found in a patient, the practitioner should prioritise sound clinical reasoning and exercise utmost caution, so that the patient is not placed at risk of an undue adverse event following LSM.

**Table 11.5 Red flags for serious pathology in the lumbar spine**

| Condition | Signs and symptoms |
|---|---|
| Cauda equina | • Urinary incontinence or loss of bladder control<br>• Bowel incontinence or lack of control over defecation<br>• Saddle (perianal/perineal) anaesthesia or paraesthesia<br>• Progressive motor weakness in the lower extremities |
| Possible cancer | • Greater than 55 years of age<br>• Past history of cancer<br>• Unexplained weight loss<br>• Constant, progressive back pain at night or at rest |
| Possible infection | • Fever, chills<br>• Recent urinary tract or skin infection<br>• Penetrating wound near spine<br>• Unrelenting night pain or pain at rest<br>• Substance abuse, intravenous drug use<br>• No improvement after six weeks of conventional treatment |

| | |
|---|---|
| Possible inflammatory disorders | • Gradual onset of symptoms<br>• Family history<br>• Morning stiffness for longer than 45 minutes<br>• Persisting limitation of movements in all directions<br>• Iritis, colitis, skin rashes, urethral discharge |
| Other possible serious spinal pathology | • Systemically unwell<br>• Widespread neuropathic pain<br>• History of significant trauma, such as a fall from a height<br>• History of trivial trauma and severe pain in potential osteoporotic individual<br>• Sudden onset of severe central pain causing patient to 'freeze' |

Sources: Nachemson and Vingard (2000); McKenzie and May (2003)

## Special Tests

### Table 11.6 Special tests for assessing serious pathology in the lumbar spine

| Test | Procedure | Positive sign | Interpretation |
|---|---|---|---|
| Straight leg raising test | The patient lies supine. The examiner lifts the patient's leg off the table while maintaining the knee in a fully extended position. The examiner continues to elevate the leg until maximum hip flexion is reached or the patient requests to stop due to pain or tightness in the back or leg. The examiner notes the angle formed between the lower limb and the examination table. The same procedure is then repeated with the opposite leg. | • Reduced angle of hip flexion, and shooting pain radiating from the lower back down to the posterior thigh | ☐ Nerve root irritation |

| Test | Procedure | Positive sign | Interpretation |
|---|---|---|---|
| Lumbar quadrant test | The patient stands before the examiner and extends the spine as far as possible. The examiner stabilises the ilium (largest bone of the pelvis) with one hand and grabs the shoulder with the other hand. The examiner then applies overpressure and leads the patient to extension while the patient laterally flexes and rotates to the side of pain. The examiner holds this position for three seconds. | • Pain, numbness or tingling in the area of the back or lower limb | ☐ Localised pain is suggestive of facet syndrome ☐ Radiating pain into the leg indicates nerve root irritation |
| Slump test | The patient sits on the edge of a treatment table, with legs supported, hands behind back and hips in neutral. The patient is then asked to slump, allowing the thoracic and lumbar spines to collapse into flexion while still looking straight ahead. The patient then flexes the neck by placing the chin on the chest and the examiner maintains the overpressure. The patient is then instructed to extend one knee as much as possible and at the same time the examiner dorsiflexes the ankle. The patient informs the examiner at each step during the procedure about what is being felt. | • Reproduction of radicular pain in the back or lower limb | ☐ Increased sciatic nerve root tension |

Sources: Phillips, Reider and Mehta (2005); Magee (2014); Majlesi *et al.* (2008); Baxter (2003); Stuber *et al.* (2014); Maitland (1985)

# References

Baxter, R.E. (2003). *Pocket Guide to Musculoskeletal Assessment*. St Louis, MO: W.B. Saunders.

Cleland, J.A., Fritz, J.M., Whitman, J.M., Childs, J.D. and Palmer, J.A. (2006). The use of a lumbar spine manipulation technique by physical therapists in patients who satisfy a clinical prediction rule: A case series. *Journal of Orthopaedic and Sports Physical Therapy, 36*(4), 209–214.

Dunn, I.F., Proctor, M.R. and Day, A.L. (2006). Lumbar spine injuries in athletes. *Neurosurgical Focus, 21*(4), 1–5.

Hansen, L., De Zee, M., Rasmussen, J., Andersen, T.B., Wong, C. and Simonsen, E.B. (2006). Anatomy and biomechanics of the back muscles in the lumbar spine with reference to biomechanical modeling. *Spine, 31*(17), 1888–1899.

Kishner, S., Moradian, M. and Morello, J.K. (2014). Lumbar spine anatomy. Medscape. Available at http://emedicine.medscape.com/article/1899031-overview (accessed 25 July 2016).

Magee, D.J. (2014). *Orthopedic Physical Assessment*. St Louis, MO: Elsevier Health Sciences.

Maitland, G.D. (1985). The slump test: Examination and treatment. *Australian Journal of Physiotherapy, 31*(6), 215–219.

Majlesi, J., Togay, H., Ünalan, H. and Toprak, S. (2008). The sensitivity and specificity of the slump and the straight leg raising tests in patients with lumbar disc herniation. *Journal of Clinical Rheumatology, 14*(2), 87–91.

McKenzie, R. and May, S. (2003). *The Lumbar Spine: Mechanical Diagnosis and Therapy*. Windham, NH: Orthopedic Physical Therapy Products.

Nachemson, A. and Vingard, E. (2000). Assessment of patients with neck and back pain: A best evidence synthesis. In A.L. Nachemson and E. Jonsson (Eds), *Neck and Back Pain: The Scientific Evidence of Causes, Diagnosis, and Treatment*. Philadelphia, PA: Lippincott Williams & Wilkins.

Oliphant, D. (2004). Safety of spinal manipulation in the treatment of lumbar disk herniations: A systematic review and risk assessment. *Journal of Manipulative and Physiological Therapeutics, 27*(3), 197–210.

Ombregt, L. (2013). *Clinical Examination of the Thoracic Spine: A System of Orthopaedic Medicine*. St Louis, MO: Elsevier Health Sciences.

OpenStax College. (2013). *Anatomy and Physiology*. Rice University.

Pearcy, M.J. and Tibrewal, S.B. (1984). Axial rotation and lateral bending in the normal lumbar spine measured by three-dimensional radiography. *Spine, 9*(6), 582–587.

Pearcy, M., Portek, I.A.N. and Shepherd, J. (1984). Three-dimensional x-ray analysis of normal movement in the lumbar spine. *Spine, 9*(3), 294–297.

Phillips, F.M., Reider, B. and Mehta, V. (2005). Lumbar spine. In B. Reider (Ed.), *The Orthopaedic Physical Examination*, 2nd edition. Philadelphia, PA: Elsevier Saunders.

Standring, S. (2008). *Gray's Anatomy: The Anatomical Basis of Clinical Practice*. London: Churchill Livingstone.

Stuber, K., Lerede, C., Kristmanson, K., Sajko, S. and Bruno, P. (2014). The diagnostic accuracy of the Kemp's test: A systematic review. *The Journal of the Canadian Chiropractic Association, 58*(3), 258.

Watson, C., Paxinos, G. and Kayalioglu, G. (Eds) (2009). *The Spinal Cord: A Christopher and Dana Reeve Foundation Text and Atlas*. London: Academic Press.

# Techniques for the Lumbar Spine

## Lumbar Roll Manipulation

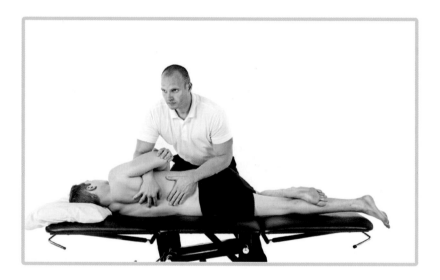

**General Set-up for a Lumbar Roll Manipulation**
- Ask the patient to lie on their side with affected side up.
- The head is in a neutral position supported using a pillow; the spine is straight with no rotation.
- The bottom leg on the table is straight, the top leg is bent with a 90-degree position at the hip, and the foot rests in the popliteal crease of the bottom knee. The patient should have their arms in a folded position in front of their chest.
- The practitioner stands at the side of the table, facing the patient.
- You will need an asymmetrical stance with a slight bias towards the head of the table.
- Hold the lower arm of the patient via their tricep and lock their wrist against your ribs.

- Slightly squat, and as you stand up pull the patient up and round. You will know when have engaged the required segment as you palpate minimal rotation of the spinous process.
- You will aim to contact the patient via the arm flexors on to the PSIS of the affected side in order to induce rotation of the lumbar spine.
- Your other hand will contact over the ribs and into the axilla via your arm flexors.
- Ask the patient to inhale and exhale.
- At the end of exhalation, engage the barrier by inducing rotation towards you via the pelvis and rotation away from you via the shoulder.
- At the barrier, complete the manipulation.

## Lumbar Roll Manipulation T12/L1

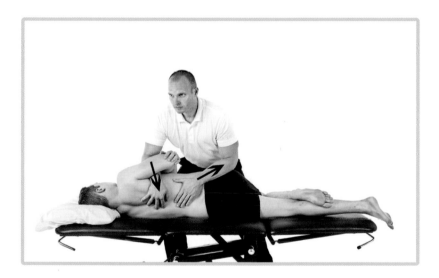

- The practitioner asks the patient to lift their top arm up slightly, allowing the practitioner's dominant arm to slide in between the patient's body and their upper arm. The practitioner's dominant hand should contact the lateral surface of the superior spinous process (T12), using the second and third fingers. The rest of the hand simply rests in a neutral position against the patient.

- The practitioner's forearm will be over the patient's rib cage and angled slightly oblique towards the patient's axilla. This pushes the patient's shoulder slightly posterior and allows the inferior to superior movement needed at the upper part of the target segment. It essentially helps encourage a counter-rotation component to the lower body. Have the patient clamp their arm down on to your arm to aid with positioning and tension.
- The practitioner's supporting hand will contact the SP of the inferior segment (L1) using the second and third fingers. The hand will be pointing towards the floor, resting on the patient's back. The forearm will be contacting over the patient's upper facing pelvic wing and on to the gluteal muscles. The practitioner's arm should be tucked in tight to their body, the elbow in by their rib cage.
- While adding minimal contact pressure on the patient's ribs and glutes, ask them to inhale.
- As the patient inhales, move your body weight up and over/across the patient so your centre of gravity point (sternal notch) is over the target segment.

## Key Points

- For patient comfort, you may want to put a towel under their top arm/over the ribs.
- Be very gentle with your contacts and do not press down. This is directly over the patient's ribs and glutes, which can be very tender and uncomfortable for the patient.
- Female practitioners – your centre of gravity is lower than males, more towards the xiphoid process, so you will need to move yourself accordingly so this is over the target segment.
- Ensure there is a breathing cycle. This allows the patient to relax and makes the manipulation more comfortable for the patient and practitioner. The thrust should only be applied at the end of the exhalation phase, when maximum tension has been released.

# Lumbar Roll Manipulation L2 to L5/S1

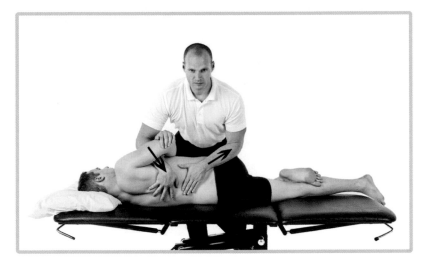

- Ask the patient to lie on their side.
- Place the patient on the side opposite the rotational restriction. They should be in a straight-line position with their body. The head is in a neutral position, supported with a pillow, the spine is straight with no rotation, the bottom leg on the table is straight, the top leg is bent with a 90-degree position at the hip, and the foot rests in the popliteal crease of the bottom knee. The patient should have their arms in a folded position in front of their chest.
- The practitioner stands at the side of the table, at a 45-degree angle to the patient.
- This is a wide asymmetrical stance with slight rotation of the front/lead leg forward towards the patient's head, the inner part of the practitioner's leg in contact with the table. The practitioner's back leg is approximately at the patient's hip level, with the outer aspect of the leg in contact with the table.
- Locate the target segment.
- Using the extensor aspect of your forearm, add rotation of the pelvis via the PSIS. Using the extensor aspect will give a broad, soft contact.
- Your other arm is in contact with the rib and axilla, again with the extensor aspect of your forearm as shown.
- Ask the patient to inhale and exhale.
- At the end of exhalation engage the barrier and complete the manipulation.

171

## Modifications to Lumbar Roll Manipulation

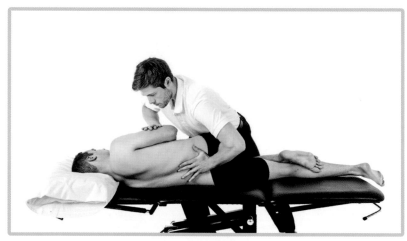

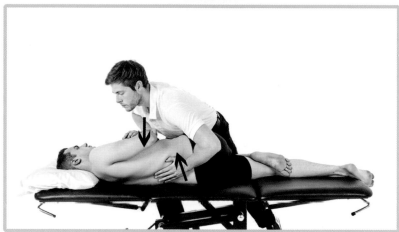

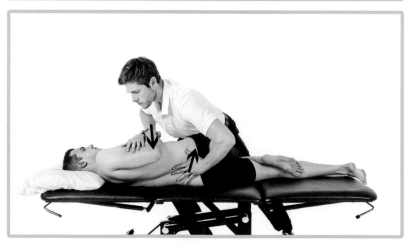

- The contact of the practitioner is slightly different to the standard lumbar role. Take note of the different arm position of the patient and practitioner.
- The contact hand should be on the mammillary process of the inferior vertebra on the side of rotational restriction, using a hypothenar (pisiform) contact. The fingers should be resting parallel to the patient's spine.
- The practitioner's support hand should contact the patient's upper forearm.
- Create pre-tension at the target segment.
- Your contact on the patient's forearm should bring the folded arms downwards and posterior.
- No downward pressure is applied here; the upper body will be glided posterior to create a counter-rotation force to the lower body during the thrust phase.
- The angulation of the patient's hip will dictate the level at which tension is achieved in the lumbar spine. The more acute the angle, the higher in the lumbar spine tension is achieved. Feel for increasing tension towards your target joint in the patient's spine by moving the patient's knee with your thigh sandwich.
- While adding minimal contact pressure on the patient, ask them to inhale.
- As the patient inhales, move your body weight up and over the patient so your centre of gravity point (sternal notch) is over the target segment.
- Your back leg comes off the ground, allowing the patient's knee to slide down between your thighs, still keeping contact with the knee as this controls the patient's rotation towards you.

## Patient's Leg Off the Table

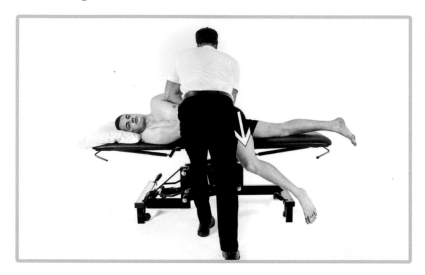

- It may not be possible for the patient to flex their top leg and bend their knee to rest in the popliteal crease of the bottom leg.
- This could be due to a hip replacement, knee replacement or osteoarthritis in the hip or knee. This technique is performed in exactly the same way as previously described.

### Key Points

- Due to the patient's leg being off the table, you will need to make sure you help them back to the supine position once you have completed the manipulation.

## Lumbar Roll Kick-Start Manipulation L2 to L5/S1

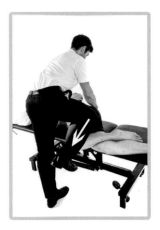 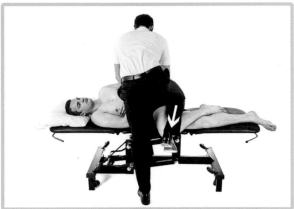

A kick start can be used as an alternative to the modified lumbar roll. It is a great way to achieve maximum power with minimal effort from the practitioner.

Female practitioners in particular love this alternative set-up, especially if they are smaller than their patient, or if they feel weak in their upper/lower body and need an extra bit of leverage to achieve the manipulation.

The initial set up of the patient is the same as for all lumbar roll techniques.

- As the patient inhales, your back leg comes off the ground; your knee fits into the patient's popliteal crease and rests here.
- As the patient exhales, you bring your knee down, causing rotation of the patient's lower body towards you to engage the barrier as the dysfunctional segment.
- Once you have engaged the barrier, perform a kick down to the floor.
- The kick-start movement happens at the practitioner's knee and is like jump-starting a motor bike (hence the name kick start).

### Key Points

- Be aware that this technique can be quite powerful as you are using very strong muscles to help with the rotation.
- Female practitioners – your centre of gravity is lower than males, more towards the xiphoid process, so you will need to move yourself accordingly so this is over the target segment.

- Ensure there is a breathing cycle. This allows the patient to relax and makes the manipulation more comfortable for the patient and practitioner. The thrust should only be applied at the end of the exhalation phase, when maximum tension has been released.
- Imagine the spine as a twisted ribbon. You want counter-rotation so that the point of tension between the upper and lower body (the target segment) is where you would imagine the twist of the ribbon to be.
- You can apply the same technique down into the SI joints and sacrum by changing your contact to the appropriate bony landmarks and by reducing the angle of flexion at the patient's hip. The lower in the lumbar spine you go, the less flexion at the patient's hip is required.
- For increased specificity, a lumbar spinous hook (push/pull) technique can be used (see the picture below). This is the same set-up as the Lumbar Roll Manipulation (see description earlier). A kick-start modification is also being used in this set-up.

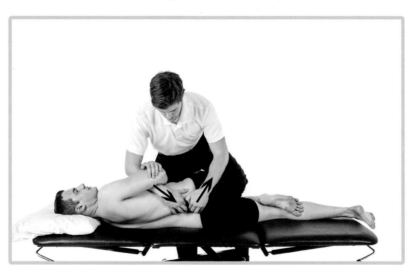

# Modified Lumbar Roll Manipulation

This technique can be used for SI joint manipulation as well as lumbar manipulation.

Alternatively, you may choose this technique for a patient with a hip or knee pathology to avoid excessive flexion in both joints.

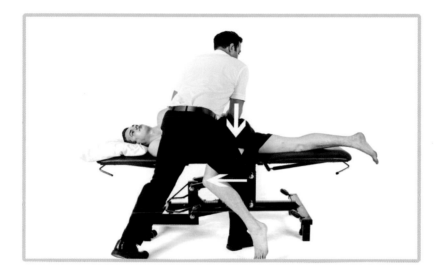

- With the patient in the side posture, rotate them as you would for lumbar manipulation for L5/S1 and allow their top leg to come off the table as shown.
- Your contact will be on the up-facing SI joint. This can be taken via a pisiform contact on the PSIS or with the forearm (flexors) of the contact hand on the PSIS.
- The support hand contacts the patient's upper forearms, as they are crossed in front of their chest.
- There will be the counter-rotation force applied posterior (away from the practitioner) here as the lower body will be rotated towards the practitioner.

- The practitioner is angled at 45 degrees to the patient in an asymmetrical stance as shown.
- The practitioner's leading leg will contact the patients popliteal space, while the practitioner's supporting leg remains in the split stance with the front of the foot contacting the floor.
- Tension at the SI joint will be controlled by the practitioner's leg slowly flexing the patient's leg superior (towards their head). There should be minimal flexion needed as a 90-degree position at the hip is sufficient for SI joint tension.
- Increasing the hip flexion further via the leg being flexed will bring tension up into the lumbar spine.
- On exhalation, perform the manipulation along the line of the femur as shown.

### Key Points

- Remember this is not about using excessive force. Speed and waiting for full exhalation is essential.
- Allow the patient to bend their knee a little in this technique to avoid neural tethering.

# Reverse Lumbar Roll

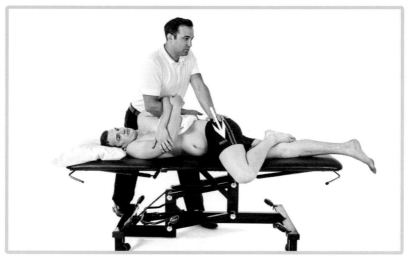

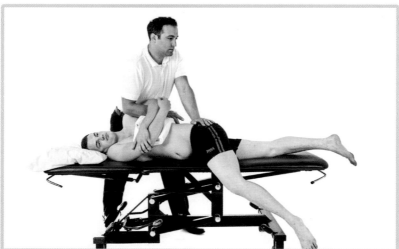

- Ask the patient to lie on their side.
- They should be in a straight-line position with their body. The head is in a neutral position, supported with a pillow; the spine is straight with no rotation.
- The bottom leg on the table is straight, the top leg is bent with a 90-degree position at the hip and the foot rests in the popliteal crease of the bottom knee.
- The patient should have their arms in a folded position in front of their chest.

179

- The practitioner stands behind the patient with an asymmetrical stance.
- Place your support arm under the patient's folded arms. This will be over the patient's anterior shoulder and ribs, so a towel may be used to make the contact more comfortable for the patient. The patient will add a bit of downward pressure on to your support arm on the exhalation phase of the manipulation.
- Alternatively, the practitioner's support hand can contact over the anterior aspect of the patient's shoulder. Ensure you are not over the glenohumeral joint directly as this can be painful for the patient. The hand is placed over the patient's upper pectoral region; a towel can be placed over this area to make the contact more comfortable.
- The practitioner's contact hand is placed over posterior aspect of the greater trochanter of the patient's top leg.
- Pre-tension in the target joint is created via rotation of the lumbar spine along the line of the femur.
- The patient's lower body is rotated anterior while the upper body/shoulder is rotated posterior. There should be equal rotation in both aspects to ensure maximum tension at the target joint. The practitioner must keep their contact arm straight with minimal bending at the elbow.
- Longitudinal/traction tension is needed to gain the barrier of the target joint. This is achieved by the practitioner already being in an asymmetrical stance with a straight contact arm, moving your body weight over the patient.
- The manipulation follows the patient's breathing..
- Do not add a body drop to the manipulation as this may impact the patient's shoulder.

### Modification

- The patient's top leg can be placed straight out in front of them, instead of in the bent 90-degree position. This can be more comfortable and practical for patients with conditions such as hip/knee osteoarthritis or joint replacements.
- The straightening of the patient's leg creates a longer lever for the practitioner, so take this into account when feeling for the barrier in the target joint.

# CHAPTER 12

# The Pelvis and Sacroiliac Joint

## Introduction

From the 19th century onwards, the use of manipulation to balance the bones and soft-tissue structures of pelvis and sacrum regions has increased progressively (Lee, 2004). Today, a variety of manipulative procedures are used as a first-line treatment for lower back, hip, pelvic and buttock pain that radiates from the lower extremity, specifically the pelvic bones and the sacroiliac joint (Laslett, 2008). Practitioners of manual therapy believe that a great majority of patients can be made immediately pain-free by applying manipulation. They claim that this can be achieved following a simple manual correction of abnormalities in the pelvic and sacrum regions, such as a perceived anterior rotary subluxation of the ilium or a nerve entrapment due ligamentous injury in the pelvis (DonTigny, 2007).

The therapeutic goal of these practitioners is to apply a procedure that is well tolerated by the recipient and yields the best result. They primarily aim at addressing any specific dysfunctions in the region, restoring mobility and function by adjusting malalignment of bony and soft-tissue structures, and strengthening the surrounding muscles (Childs *et al.*, 2004). In addition, they usually utilise two general manipulation approaches for manual correction of pelvic and sacroiliac abnormalities: high-velocity, low-amplitude thrust (HVLAT) and low-velocity, low-amplitude thrust.

However, manipulation should be avoided if an absolute contraindication or a red flag for serious pathology is identified (Rivett, Thomas and Bolton, 2005). Appropriate care should be taken if a relative contraindication to manipulation is present, so that the patient is not exposed to an undue risk of injury. Furthermore, because adequate knowledge and skill, extensive experience and sound clinical reasoning play an important part in preventing incidence of adverse events following manipulation, practitioners should have an appropriate training and education before they start applying manipulative procedures to their patients (World Health Organization, 2005; Ernst, 2007).

Therefore, this chapter is written to describe the various joints of the pelvis and sacrum, the range of motion in these joints and appropriate special tests to diagnose serious pathology in the regions. In addition, this chapter will also describe some of the common injuries to the pelvis and sacrum, and the red flags for manipulation.

## Joints

In human anatomy, the pelvis is interposed between the lower spinal column and the lower extremities. It includes the pelvic girdle (the two coxal bones), the sacrum and the coccyx. Each coxal bone results from a fusion of three bones – the ilium, the ischium, and the pubis – and is firmly attached to the axial skeleton because of its articulation with the sacrum, the sacroiliac joint (McCann and Wise, 2014). The pelvis is divided into the false and true pelvis separated by an oblique line known as the pelvic brim. The pelvis functions as the site of attachment for the lower limbs. It also protects the internal reproductive organs, the urinary bladder and a portion of the large intestine (OpenStax, 2013; Standring, 2008).

**Table 12.1 The joints of the pelvis and sacrum**

| Joint name | Description | Function |
|---|---|---|
| Acetabulofemoral joint | • A synovial, ball-and-socket joint formed by joining the head of the femur with the acetabulum of the pelvis<br>• Involves articulation between the lower limb and the pelvic girdle<br>• Responsible for linking the lower extremity with the axial skeleton of the trunk and pelvis<br>• Also known as the hip joint | • Supports the body weight in both dynamic and static postures<br>• Helps to maintain the balance of the body |

| | | |
|---|---|---|
| Sacroiliac joint | <ul><li>A true diarthrodial joint that is characteristically different to other diarthrodial joints</li><li>Involves articulation between the sacrum and the pelvis (ilium bones)</li><li>Usually formed within the sacral segments of S1, S2 and S3</li><li>Has fibrocartilage in addition to hyaline cartilage</li><li>Is a less mobile, well-innervated joint and is therefore very strong and stable</li></ul> | <ul><li>Serves as shock absorber for the spine</li><li>Helps transmit the weight of the upper extremity to the pelvis and legs</li><li>Provides stability to the spine and pelvis</li><li>Helps to maintain the body balance during walking (push-off phase)</li></ul> |
| Lumbosacral joint | <ul><li>A cartilaginous, multifunctional joint that connects the lumbar spine with the sacrum</li><li>Involves articulation between the vertebral bodies of the last lumbar vertebra (L5) and the first sacral segment (S1)</li><li>Consists of several interconnected components, including a disc between the two articulating vertebral bodies and two facet joints</li></ul> | <ul><li>Provides a strong and stable base for the vertebral column</li><li>Permits the trunk of the body to twist and bend in almost all directions</li></ul> |

Sources: Cereatti *et al.* (2010); Forst *et al.* (2006); Vleeming *et al.* (2012); Lin *et al.* (2001)

## Range of Motion

The hip muscles exert three degrees of freedom on three mutually perpendicular axes. These movements include the transverse axis (flexion and extension), the longitudinal axis (lateral and medial rotation) and the sagittal axis (abduction and adduction) (Schünke *et al.*, 2006). A substantial motion, in fact, takes place at the external pelvic platform. Movement of the pelvis upon the hip joints is relative to the femur. Coupled movement of the hip and pelvis plays a significant role in establishing lordosis and kyphosis in the lower spine (Vleeming and Stoeckart, 2007).

**Table 12.2 Estimated normal range of motion of the hip**

| Movement type | Range of motion |
|---|---|
| Flexion | 115–125° |
| Extension | 0–15° |
| Abduction | 30–50° |
| Adduction | 30° |
| Lateral Rotation | 30–40° |
| Medial Rotation | 40–60° |

Source: Seidenberg and Childress (2005)

In contrast, the range of motion in the sacroiliac joint is small (Forst *et al.*, 2006). Although the medical community has for years held fast to the notion that the joint is motionless, except in the presence of disease or pregnancy, several empirical studies have demonstrated presence of a screw-axis motion at the sagittal plane of the joint (Fortin, 1993; Sturesson, Selvik and Udén, 1989; Sturesson, Uden and Vleeming, 2000).

## Range of Motion at the Sacroiliac Joint

- Less than 4° of rotation
- Up to 1.6mm of translation

Source: Adapted from Sturesson *et al.* (1989, 2000)

## Common Injuries

A major injury to the pelvis and the sacrum is often caused by a fall, motor vehicle accident, violent activity or sports trauma. These injuries are common in all populations, including male and female, the very young and the old, and participants of numerous sports (Larkin, 2010).

**Table 12.3 Common injuries to the pelvis and sacrum**

| Injury | Characteristics |
|---|---|
| Pelvic fracture | • A break of one or more bony structures of the pelvis, including the hip bone, sacrum, and coccyx<br>• Often caused by some type of traumatic, high-energy event, such as falls from height, motor vehicle accidents or crush injuries<br>• Severity range from low-energy, relatively benign injuries to high-energy, life-threatening fractures<br>• Represent 3% of all skeletal fractures in the United States |
| Sacroiliac joint dysfunction | • Generally refers to pain or discomfort arising the sacroiliac joint structures<br>• Characterised as aberrant position or abnormal motion in the region, either too little or too much<br>• Often results from some type of traumatic event, such as a direct fall on the buttocks, motor vehicle accident or a step into an unexpected hole<br>• Common symptoms include lower back pain, buttock pain, hip pain, groin pain, sciatic leg pain, frequent urination and transient numbness |
| Hip dislocation | • Usually results from a traumatic injury, a high energy directed along the axis of the femur<br>• Can be anterior, posterior or central<br>• May occur with associated injuries, such as fractures of the femoral head or neck<br>• Often occurs because of motor vehicle accidents (about 70% of cases)<br>• Occurs predominantly in the posterior region (about 90% of cases) |

Sources: Furey *et al.* (2009); Langford *et al.* (2013); Laslett (2008); Fortin (1993); Vleeming *et al.* (2012); Kovacevic, Mariscalco and Goodwin (2011); Seidenberg (2010)

# Red Flags

Red flags help to identify serious pathology in patients with chronic pain. If a red flag symptom is found in a patient, the practitioner should prioritise sound clinical reasoning and exercise utmost caution, so that the patient is not placed at risk of an undue adverse event due to manipulation.

**Table 12.4 Red flags for serious pathology in the pelvis and sacrum**

| Condition | Signs and symptoms |
|---|---|
| Pathological fractures of the femoral neck | • Older females over 70 years of age<br>• Severe, constant hip, groin or knee pain<br>• Past history of trauma such as a fall from a standing position |
| Avascular necrosis (AVN) of the femoral head | • Prolonged corticosteroid use<br>• History of excessive alcohol use<br>• History of slipped capital femoral epiphysis<br>• Gradual onset of pain<br>• Groin, thigh or medial knee pain – worse with weight bearing |
| Cancer | • Previous history of cancer (e.g. prostate, breast or any reproductive cancer)<br>• Unexpected loss of weight<br>• Constant, progressive pain unchanged by positions or movement |
| Colon cancer | • Age over 50 years<br>• Family history of colon cancer<br>• Bowel disturbances (e.g. rectal bleeding, black stools) |
| Infection | • Fever, chills<br>• Recent urinary tract or skin infection<br>• Burning sensation with urination<br>• Unrelenting night pain or pain at rest<br>• No improvement after six weeks of conventional treatment |

Sources: Reiman and Thorborg (2014); Gabbe *et al.* (2009); Henschke, Maher and Refshauge (2007); Meyers *et al.* (2000); Van den Bruel *et al.* (2010)

## Special Tests

### Table 12.5 Special tests for assessing serious pathology in the pelvis and sacrum

| Test | Procedure | Positive sign | Interpretation |
|------|-----------|---------------|----------------|
| Trendelen-burg's sign | The patient stands on both feet. The examiner asks the patient to slowly raise one foot off the ground, without taking any additional support. The patient keeps an upright posture without significant tilt of the upper trunk. | • A compensatory tilt of the torso or a drop of the contralateral iliac crest | ☐ Presence of a muscular dysfunction<br>☐ Subluxation or dislocation of the hip |
| Faber's test | The patient lies supine and the tested leg is placed in a flexed, abducted, externally rotated position. | • Pain elicited on the ipsilateral side anteriorly | ☐ Hip joint disorder |
| | | • Pain elicited on the contralateral side posteriorly | ☐ Sacroiliac joint dysfunction |
| Gaenslen's test | The patient lies either supine or in a side-lying position. The examiner instructs the patient to draw both the legs up to the chest. The patient then slowly lowers the test leg into extension. | • Pain in the sacroiliac joint | ☐ Sacroiliac joint dysfunction |
| Ober's test | The patient is placed in a lateral decubitus position. The affected knee is then flexed to 90° while pelvis is stabilised. The examiner passively abducts and pulls the patient's upper leg posteriorly until the thigh is in line with the torso. | • Leg remains abducted and does not fall to the table | ☐ Excessive tightness of the iliotibial band |

| Test | Procedure | Positive sign | Interpretation |
|------|-----------|---------------|----------------|
| Thomas test | The patient lies supine with the back flat on the table. The patient is then instructed to flex one leg and pull it to the chest with their hands. | • Straight leg lifting off of the exam table | ☐ Flexion contracture of the hip |
| Log roll test | The patient lies supine with both hip and knee extended. The examiner passively rotates both fully extended legs internally and externally. | • Pain in the anterior hip or groin | ☐ Piriformis syndrome<br>☐ Slipped capital femoral epiphysis |
| Ely's test | The patient lies prone with legs fully extended. The examiner passively flexes the knee, making the heel touch the buttock. The examiner then observes the ipsilateral hip for vertical separation from the exam table. | • Hip is forced to lift off of the exam table | ☐ Rectus femoris contracture |

Sources: Baxter (2003); McRae (2010); McFadden and Seidenberg (2010)

# References

Baxter, R.E. (2003). *Pocket Guide to Musculoskeletal Assessment*. St Louis, MO: W.B. Saunders.

Cereatti, A., Margheritini, F., Donati, M. and Cappozzo, A. (2010). Is the human acetabulofemoral joint spherical? *Bone and Joint Journal, 92*(2), 311–314.

Childs, J.D., Fritz, J.M., Flynn, T.W., Irrgang, J.J. *et al.* (2004). A clinical prediction rule to identify patients with low back pain most likely to benefit from spinal manipulation: A validation study. *Annals of Internal Medicine, 141*(12), 920–928.

DonTigny, R.L. (2007). A detailed and critical biomechanical analysis of the sacroiliac joints and relevant kinesiology. The implications for lumbopelvic function and dysfunction. In A. Vleeming, V. Mooney and R. Stoeckart (Eds), *Movement, Stability and Lumbopelvic Pain: Integration of Research and Therapy*, 2nd edition, London: Churchill Livingstone.

Ernst, E. (2007). Adverse effects of spinal manipulation: A systematic review. *Journal of the Royal Society of Medicine, 100*(7), 330–338.

Forst, S.L., Wheeler, M.T., Fortin, J.D. and Vilensky, J.A. (2006). The sacroiliac joint: Anatomy, physiology and clinical significance. *Pain Physician, 9*(1), 61–67.

Fortin, J.D. (1993). Sacroiliac Joint: A new perspective. *Journal of Back and Musculoskeletal Rehabilitation, 3*(3), 31–43.

Furey, A.J., Toole, R.V., Nascone, J.W., Sciadini, M.F., Copeland, C.E. and Turen, C. (2009). Classification of pelvic fractures: Analysis of inter-and intraobserver variability using the Young-Burgess and Tile classification systems. *Orthopedics, 32*(6), 401.

Gabbe, B.J., Bailey, M., Cook, J.L., Makdissi, M. *et al.* (2009). The association between hip and groin injuries in the elite junior football years and injuries sustained during elite senior competition. *British Journal of Sports Medicine, 44*(1), 799–802.

Henschke, N., Maher, C.G. and Refshauge, K.M. (2007). Screening for malignancy in low back pain patients: A systematic review. *European Spine Journal, 16*(10), 1673–1679.

Kovacevic, D., Mariscalco, M. and Goodwin, R.C. (2011). Injuries about the hip in the adolescent athlete. *Sports Medicine and Arthroscopy Review, 19*(1), 64–74.

Langford, J.R., Burgess, A.R., Liporace, F.A. and Haidukewych, G.J. (2013). Pelvic fractures: Part 1. Evaluation, classification, and resuscitation. *Journal of the American Academy of Orthopaedic Surgeons, 21*(8), 448–457.

Larkin, B. (2010). Epidemiology of hip and pelvis injury. In: *The Hip and Pelvis in Sports Medicine and Primary Care.* New York, NY: Springer.

Laslett, M. (2008). Evidence-based diagnosis and treatment of the painful sacroiliac joint. *Journal of Manual and Manipulative Therapy, 16*(3), 142–152.

Lee, D.G. (2004). *The Pelvic Girdle,* 3rd edition. Edinburgh: Elsevier.

Lin, Y.H., Chen, C.S., Cheng, C.K., Chen, Y.H., Lee, C.L. and Chen, W.J. (2001). Geometric parameters of the in vivo tissues at the lumbosacral joint of young Asian adults. *Spine, 26*(21), 2362–2367.

McCann, S. and Wise, E. (2014). *Kaplan Anatomy Coloring Book.* New York, NY: Kaplan Publishing.

McFadden, D.P. and Seidenberg, P.H. (2010). Physical examination of the hip and pelvis. In: *The Hip and Pelvis in Sports Medicine and Primary Care.* New York, NY: Springer.

McRae, R. (2010). *Clinical Orthopaedic Examination.* Edinburgh: Elsevier.

Meyers, W.C., Foley, D.P., Garrett, W.E., Lohnes, J.H. and Mandlebaum, B.R. (2000). Management of severe lower abdominal or inguinal pain in high-performance athletes. *American Journal of Sports Medicine, 28*(1), 2–8.

OpenStax College. (2013). *Anatomy and Physiology.* Houston, TX: Rice University.

Reiman, M.P. and Thorborg, K. (2014) Invited clinical commentary. Clinical examination and physical assessment of hip joint-related pain in athletes. *International Journal of Sports Physical Therapy, 9*(6), 737–755.

Rivett, D.A., Thomas, L. and Bolton, B. (2005). Premanipulative testing: Where do we go from here? *New Zealand Journal of Physiotherapy, 33*(3), 78–84.

Schünke, M., Ross, L.M., Schulte, E., Schumacher, U. and Lamperti, E.D. (2006.) *Thieme Atlas of Anatomy: General Anatomy and Musculoskeletal System.* New York, NY: Thieme Medical Publishers.

Seidenberg, P.H. and Childress, M.A. (2005). Evaluating hip pain in athletes. *Journal of Musculoskeletal Medicine, 22*(5), 246–254.

Seidenberg, P.H. (2010). Adult hip and pelvis disorders. In: *The Hip and Pelvis in Sports Medicine and Primary Care.* New York, NY: Springer.

Standring, S. (2008). *Gray's Anatomy: The Anatomical Basis of Clinical Practice*. London: Churchill Livingstone.

Sturesson, B., Selvik, G. and Udén, A. (1989). Movements of the sacroiliac joints: A Roentgen stereophotogrammetric analysis. *Spine, 14*(2), 162–165.

Sturesson, B., Uden, A. and Vleeming, A. (2000). A radiostereometric analysis of the movements of the sacroiliac joints in the reciprocal straddle position. *Spine, 25*(2), 214.

Van den Bruel, A., Haj-Hassan, T., Thompson, M., Buntinx, F., Mant, D. and European Research Network on Recognising Serious Infection Investigators (2010). Diagnostic value of clinical features at presentation to identify serious infection in children in developed countries: A systematic review. *The Lancet, 375*(9717), 834–845.

Vleeming A. and Stoeckart, R. (2007). The role of the pelvic girdle in coupling the spine and the legs: A clinical-anatomical perspective on pelvic stability. In A. Vleeming, V. Mooney and R. Stoeckart (Eds), *Movement, Stability and Lumbopelvic Pain: Integration and Research*. Edinburgh: Churchill Livingstone.

Vleeming, A., Schuenke, M.D., Masi, A.T., Carreiro, J.E., Danneels, L. and Willard, F.H. (2012). The sacroiliac joint: An overview of its anatomy, function and potential clinical implications. *Journal of Anatomy, 221*(6), 537–567.

World Health Organization (2005). *WHO Guidelines on Basic Training and Safety in Chiropractic*. Geneva: World Health Organization.

# Techniques for the Pelvis and Sacroiliac Joint

## Anteriorise Ilium

- Ask your patient to lie prone.
- Stand on the patient's affected side.
- Place your forearm on both the superior aspect of the iliac crest and the PSIS.
- Place your other hand underneath the patient's thigh on the involved side and interlock your hands together.
- Using the forearm as a lever, lift the patient's thigh into extension and induce adduction until a barrier is engaged.
- Maintain PA pressure with the forearm over the PSIS and iliac crest and maintain the hip extension and adduction.
- Using your for forearm, deliver a manipulation through the PSIS.

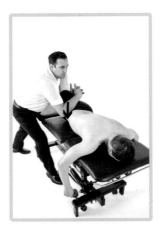

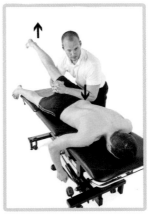

### Key Points

- A pillow can be placed under the patient's abdomen to prevent lumbar hyper extension.
- You should not perform this manipulation if there is a history of knee pathology or replacement or lumbar spine problems that may be exacerbated.
- You do not need as much extension and adduction as you may think.
- You may not hear an audible 'click' with this technique, so always retest.

# Sacroiliac Joint Manipulation – 'Chicago'

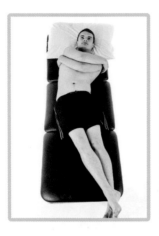 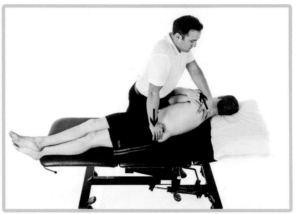

- The practitioner stands at the patient's unaffected side.
- The patient lies supine, and is placed in a bow shape. We call this 'smile away': when you are standing in the correct position, the patient's body should look as if it is smiling, not frowning.
- The legs can be placed either functional over dysfunctional or dysfunctional over functional.
- The patient's arms should be folded across the chest.
- Adopt an asymmetrical stance with your rear leg in contact with the table.
- With the heel of your dominant contact hand, contact the patient's contralateral anterior superior iliac spine (ASIS).
- With the other hand, grasp the patient's posterior shoulder, superior and lateral to the scapula.
- Ask the patient to inhale and exhale.
- Towards the end of exhalation, apply an AP and slight SI pressure through the ASIS with the heel of your hand.
- As you increase the pressure, rotate the patient's upper body towards you with your other hand until you feel the pelvis start to rotate; this occurs when you engage the barrier.
- At this point increase pressure through the heel of your hand and apply a manipulation through the ASIS.

**Key Points**

- You can incline the table to a maximum of 45 degrees to help you rotate the patient, especially if they are much bigger than you.
- Legs can be placed either dysfunctional over functional or functional over dysfunctional.
- Place a small towel over the ASIS to increase the patient's comfort.
- Always work with the patient's breathing and manipulate at the end of exhalation.

## Sacroiliac Joint Ischium Contact – Side-Lying – Posterior Innominate

- Lie the patient down on their side, with the involved side up, arms folded across chest.
- Stand on the side, facing the patient in an asymmetrical stance.
- Instruct the patient to straighten the bottom leg or help them to do it.
- Add hip and knee flexion of the leg nearest to you and tuck the foot behind the knee.
- Place your left hand on the patient's elbows (or upper arm if more appropriate) and maintain a firm pressure towards the table and superiorly to immobilise the upper body and create tension.
- Take your right hand and contact the patient's ischial tuberosity, rolling them towards you slightly. Maintain pressure on the patient's upper body so the only movement comes from the patient's lower body.
- Lean over the patient, maintaining contact with both the ischial tuberosity and the patient's arms until your sternum is over the patient's ischial tuberosity.
- Ask the patient to inhale and exhale, and engage the barrier by adding rotation to the upper body and compression to the ischium.
- Using the heel of the hand, manipulate the innominate in the PA and IS direction.
- If necessary, more tension can be created by adding an SI force through the patient's thigh using your own leg while rolling the patient towards you, further tensioning the sacroiliac joint.
- This technique moves the involved innominate in a posterior direction.

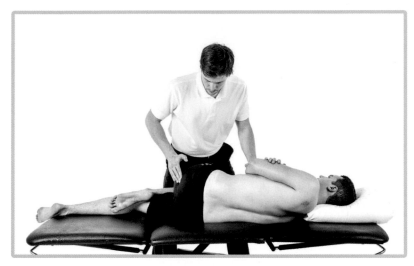

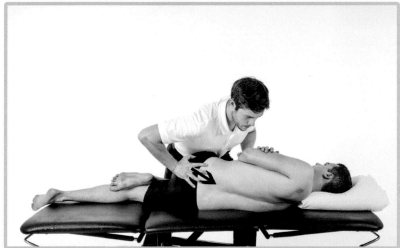

### Key Points

- You may want to place a pillow under the patient's head if using a bench without a headrest to keep the neck in neutral.
- You can place a towel over the elbows to reduce direct compression on to the wrist extensors.
- Often a patient may feel as if they are rolling off the table; reassure them this is not so in order for them to relax.
- You can also modify the Lumbar Roll Kick-Start Manipulation from the lumbar spine section in Chapter 11.
- The Modified Lumbar Roll also has a very similar effect. Again, see Chapter 11.

# Sacroiliac Joint PSIS Contact – Side Lying – Anterior Innominate

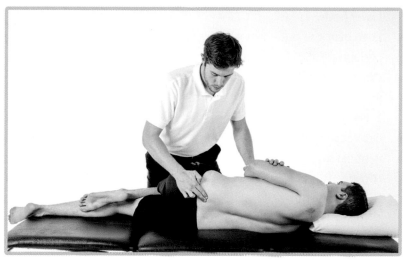

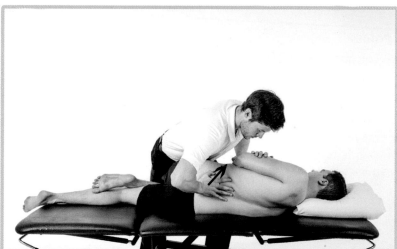

- Lie the patient down on their side, with the involved side up, arms folded across chest.
- Stand to the side, facing the patient in an asymmetrical stance.
- Instruct the patient to straighten the bottom leg or help them to do it.
- Add hip and knee flexion of the leg nearest to you and tuck the foot behind the knee.

195

- Place your caudal hand on the patient's superior pole of the PSIS and roll the patient towards you, while maintaining firm pressure through the patient's elbows to ensure the only rotation comes from the lower body.
- Lean over the patient until your sternum is over your contact on the patient's PSIS.
- With your left hand, push the upper body away. With the heel of your right hand, through the PSIS in a PA and slight IS direction push towards you to engage the barrier.
- Deliver the manipulation through the PSIS.
- If necessary, more tension can be created by adding an SI force through the patient's thigh using your own caudal leg while rolling the patient towards you, further tensioning the sacroiliac joint. If using this technique, instruct the patient that you will have thigh-to-thigh contact.
- This effectively moves the involved innominate in an anterior direction.

**Key Points**
- You may want to place a pillow under the head if using a bench without a headrest to keep the neck in neutral.
- You can place a towel over the elbows to reduce direct compression on to the wrist extensors.
- Often a patient may feel as if they are rolling off the table; reassure them this is not so in order for them to relax.
- You can also modify the Lumbar Roll Kick-Start Manipulation from the lumbar spine section in Chapter 11.
- The Modified Lumbar Roll also has a very similar effect. Again, see Chapter 11.

# The Sacral Toggle

- Ask the patient to lie prone and place a pillow under the patient's stomach to maintain a neutral lumbar spine.
- Interlace your fingers and cover the superior and inferior portion of the sacrum.

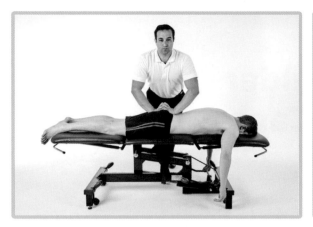

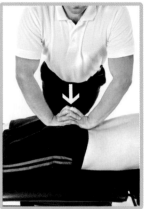

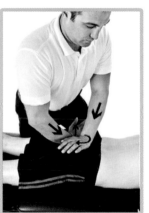

- Lean over the patient so your sternum is directly over the patient's sacrum.
- Ask the patient to inhale and exhale.
- At the midpoint of exhalation, compress the sacrum by squeezing both hands towards each other and adding slight PA pressure.
- At the end of the exhalation, add more PA pressure to engage the barrier.
- Once the barrier has been reached, add a direct manipulation PA to the sacrum.
- Quickly release your hands, releasing the tension.

**Key Points**
- This technique can be repeated 2–3 times if necessary.
- If one side is more painful or stiffer, focusing on compressing the sacrum on that side may have a greater effect as shown in the second picture.

# CHAPTER 13

# The Shoulder and Rib Cage

## Introduction

Over the past decades, high-velocity, low-amplitude thrust (HVLAT) manipulation has been an effective means to treat a variety of shoulder problems, including frozen shoulder, general shoulder pain, scapular dyskinesis, impingement syndrome, rotator cuff injury and many more. Practitioners of manipulative therapy use various techniques, depending on the shoulder joint and/or lesion being treated. They primarily aim to alleviate muscular spasm, reposition a joint subluxation and fix ligamentous retraction (Lason and Peeters, 2014).

On the other hand, manipulation of the ribs or rib cage is usually performed to treat a number of chest and rib problems, including chest pain and tightness, asthma, pneumonia, rib pain and dysfunctions, rib fracture and dislocation, and middle back pain, to name a few. Manipulative therapy practitioners use hands-on manipulation techniques to improve mobility and function in the thoracic and rib-cage region. Therapeutically, they aim at addressing any specific dysfunctions in the region and increasing the strength of the surrounding muscles (William, Glynn and Cleland, 2015).

However, before deciding to perform a manipulative technique in both the shoulder and rib cage, a practitioner must make sure that no red flags or contraindications are present (Rivett, Thomas and Bolton, 2005). In addition, because adequate knowledge, skill and experience play a key role in preventing incidence of adverse events after manipulation, it is of critical importance for manual therapy practitioners to have appropriate training and education before applying a technique (World Health Organization, 2005; Ernst, 2007). They must know how to grade various manoeuvres and when to stop.

Therefore, this chapter is written to describe the various joints of the shoulder and rib cage, the range of motion in these joints and appropriate special tests to diagnose serious pathology in the regions. In addition, this chapter will also describe some of the common injuries to the shoulder and rib cage, and the red flags for manipulation.

## Joints

The shoulder joint is one of the most complex joints in the human body. Unison of three bones – the humerus, scapula and clavicle – form this joint, connecting the upper extremity to the axial skeleton. These bones are positioned in a special harmony that allows very considerable movement of the shoulder in different stages of motion (Halder, Itoi and An, 2000). However, the shoulder joint lacks strong ligaments; for this reason, it heavily relies on the rotator cuff muscles for stability (Bigliani *et al.*, 1996).

The rib cage, in contrast, is an osteocartilaginous frame in the chest, an arrangement of bones and cartilages that encloses the chest cavity and supports the shoulder girdle and upper extremities. It is made up of 12 pairs of ribs, the sternum and the 12 thoracic vertebrae (Mader, 2004). It shields the vital organs of the body, providing attachment sites for muscles and forming a semi-rigid chamber that can expand and contract during respiration (White and Folkens, 2005).

## Table 13.1 The joints of the shoulder and rib cage

| Joint name | Description | Function |
|---|---|---|
| Glenohumeral joint | <ul><li>A multiaxial, ball-and-socket joint that is considered the most mobile in the body</li><li>Involves articulation between the humeral head and the lateral scapula</li><li>Responsible for linking the upper extremity to the trunk</li><li>Has mismatching and asymmetrical surfaces</li><li>Static stabilisers include the joint capsule, the labrum glenoidale, the articulating surfaces, the glenohumeral ligaments and the coracohumeral ligament</li></ul> | <ul><li>Allows extensive mobility for upper extremities in almost all direction</li><li>Supports a wide range of motion, including flexion, extension, lateral and medial rotation, circular rotation, abduction and adduction</li></ul> |
| Acromioclavicular joint | <ul><li>A synovial joint at the top of the shoulder</li><li>Involves articulation between the lateral end of the clavicle and the medial edge of the acromion</li><li>Covered by a fibrous capsule and strengthened by the coracoacromial ligaments (the trapezoid and conoid ligaments)</li><li>Static stabilisers include the ligaments, intra-articular disc and capsule</li></ul> | <ul><li>Serves to provide stability to the shoulder</li><li>Helps in transmitting forces between the clavicle and the acromion</li><li>Contributes to total arm movement</li></ul> |

| | | |
|---|---|---|
| Sternoclavicular joint | • A synovial double-plane joint formed by the connection of the sternum's upper portion and the clavicle's medial end<br>• Involves true articulation between the axial skeleton and the upper extremity<br>• Consists of two sections, partitioned by a complete disc or meniscus<br>• Static stabilisers include a thick capsule and supporting ligaments, such as costoclavicular, interclavicular and sternoclavicular ligaments | • Allows the clavicle to freely move in nearly all planes, allowing elevation, depression, protraction as well as retraction<br>• Provides the shoulder the ability to thrust forward |
| Costovertebral joint | • A synovial joint that connects the head of the rib with the costal facets of adjacent vertebral bodies and the intervertebral disc in between<br>• Composed of a fibrous capsule, the fan-shaped radiate ligament and the interarticular ligament | • Serves to support spinal movement<br>• Helps the ribs to work in a parallel fashion while breathing |
| Costochondral joint | • A hyaline cartilaginous joint that attaches the ribs to the costal cartilages<br>• Involves articulation between the ribs and costal cartilage | • Serves to provide stability to the rib cage |
| Costotransverse joint | • Forms when the tubercle of the rib articulates with the transverse process of the corresponding vertebra<br>• Consists of a capsule, the neck and tubercle ligaments, and the costotransverse ligaments<br>• Absent in T11 and T12 | • Helps the ribs to work in a parallel fashion while breathing |

Sources: Terry and Chopp (2000); Rockwood Jr *et al.* (2009); Van Tongel *et al.* (2012); Duprey *et al.* (2010); Palastanga and Soames (2011); Bontrager and Lampignano (2013)

## Range of Motion

The shoulder joint is the most flexible and mobile joint in the entire human body. Its movements result from a complex dynamic relationship of bony articulations, tendinous restraints, ligament constraints and dynamic muscle forces (Terry and Chopp, 2000). The shoulder joint's hyperactive mobility affords the upper extremity with a myriad range of motions, including abduction, adduction internal and external rotation, extension and flexion. In addition, the shoulder allows for scapular extension, elevation, depression and retraction (Quillen, Wuchner and Hatch, 2004). This extensive range of motion, in turn, enables the arm of the athlete to perform a versatile range of sports activities.

**Table 13.2 Normal range of motion in the shoulder**

| Motion type | Range of motion |
| --- | --- |
| Forward flexion | 180° |
| Extension | 45–60° |
| Abduction | 150° |
| Internal rotation | 70–90° |
| External rotation | 90° |

Source: Adapted from Moses (2007)

In contrast to the shoulder, the rib cage is one of the least mobile regions in the human body, although it allows required mobility for the respiratory cycle. However, this mobility is attributable to the sternal and vertebral joints and the costal cartilages at either end of the rib structure. More precisely, movements of the ribs primarily rely on the orientation of costovertebral and costotransverse joints, which are routinely subjected to continual movement (Yoganandan and Pintar, 1998). In general, the movements of the ribs are normally around two axes. The upper rib motion resembles a 'pump-handle' and the lower rib motion resembles a 'bucket-handle'. The axis for rib motion is outlined as a line running between the costovertebral joint and the costotransverse joint via the rib neck. The axis for upper rib rotation (ribs 2–6) orients towards the frontal plane, whereas the lower ribs (excluding ribs 11 and 12) lie more towards the sagittal plane (Crooper, 1996).

## Common Injuries

A major injury to the shoulder and rib cage is often caused by a fall, motor vehicle accident, violent activity, sport accident or penetrating trauma. Such injuries usually lead to a fracture, and subsequently to pain and poor functioning at the shoulder and rib-cage regions. However, the shoulder is more prone to injuries compared with the rib cage because of its hyperactive mobility (Sofu *et al.*, 2014). It is a site of many common injuries, including rotator cuff tears, frozen shoulder, tendonitis, bursitis, fractures, strains, sprains, dislocations and separations. On the other hand, although motor vehicle accident has been found to be the most common mechanism of injury for rib cage, rib fracture is one of the most common injuries to the chest, occurring in approximately 10% of all patients admitted after blunt trauma (Liman *et al.*, 2003).

**Table 13.3 Common injuries of the shoulder and rib cage**

| Injury | Characteristics |
|---|---|
| Glenohumeral dislocation | <ul><li>Occurs when the articulation between the head of the humerus and the glenoid fossa is moved out of contact</li><li>Approximately 96% of all shoulder dislocations are anterior, with the rest being posterior</li><li>The annual incidence rate is 17 per 100,000 population</li><li>Usually occurs in young and middle-aged people</li></ul> |
| Clavicle fracture | <ul><li>A common acute shoulder injury frequently caused by a fall on the lateral shoulder</li><li>Accounts for 2.6% to 5% of all fractures (about 1 in every 20 fractures) and 44% of all shoulder girdle injuries in adults</li><li>Accounts for 10% to 16% of all fractures in childhood</li><li>Affects 30–60 cases per 100,000 population globally</li><li>Occurs 2.5 times more commonly in men than in women</li></ul> |

| Injury | Characteristics |
|--------|-----------------|
| Acromioclavicular sprain | • A common injury in athletes and active persons<br>• Usually results when a direct blow or force is applied to the acromion with the humerus adducted<br>• Accounts for roughly 12% of all shoulder dislocations<br>• Affects males more commonly than females, with a ratio of around 5:1<br>• Men between their second and fourth decades of life have the highest frequency of incidence |
| Proximal humerus fracture | • A quite rare fracture and has a poor prognosis<br>• Responsible for 1% to 3% of all fractures, and roughly 20% of all fractures of the bone<br>• Annual incidence in people 16 years or older is 14.5 per 100,000, although gradually increases from the fifth decade<br>• Occurs more frequently in elderly people<br>• Usually results from a fall on to an outstretched arm |
| Rib fracture | • Often results from a direct blow to the chest, but may also occur because of coughing or forceful muscular activity of the upper limb or trunk<br>• Most frequently affects ribs 7 and 10<br>• Occurs more often in older persons than in younger adults<br>• Symptoms include severe well-localised pain, pain during deep inspiration or with movement and grating sound with breathing or movement |

Sources: Dala-Ali *et al.* (2012); Krøner, Lind and Jensen (1989); Khan *et al.* (2009); Jeray (2007); Zlowodzki *et al.* (2005); Lynch *et al.* (2013); Quillen *et al.* (2004); Ekholm *et al.* (2006); Melendez and Doty (2015); Ombregt (2003)

## Red Flags

Red flags help to identify serious pathology in patients with chronic pain. If a red flag symptom is found in a patient, the practitioner should prioritise sound clinical reasoning and exercise utmost caution, so that the patient is not placed at risk of an undue adverse event due to manipulation.

**Table 13.4 Red flags for serious pathology in the shoulder and rib cage**

| Condition | Signs and symptoms |
|---|---|
| Acute rotator cuff tear | <ul><li>Trauma</li><li>Acute disabling pain in the shoulder</li><li>Sensory deficits</li><li>Significant muscle weakness</li><li>Positive drop-arm test</li></ul> |
| Neurological lesion | <ul><li>Unexplained wasting</li><li>Significant neurological deficit (e.g. sensory or motor)</li><li>Persistent headaches</li></ul> |
| Radiculopathy | <ul><li>Severe radiating pain</li><li>Pins-and-needles sensation in shoulder</li></ul> |
| Dropped head syndrome | <ul><li>Severe neck extensor muscle weakness</li><li>Profound sparing of flexors</li><li>Chin-on-chest deformity</li><li>Neck stiffness</li><li>Weakness of shoulder girdle</li></ul> |
| Unreduced dislocation | <ul><li>Major trauma</li><li>Epileptic fit</li><li>Electric shock</li><li>Loss of rotation and normal shape</li></ul> |
| Myocardial infarction | <ul><li>Chest pain or discomfort</li><li>Pressure or tightness in the chest</li><li>Shortness of breath, sweating, pallor, tremors, lightheadedness and nausea</li><li>History of a sedentary lifestyle</li><li>Previous history of ischaemic heart disease, abnormally high blood pressure, diabetes, smoking, elevated triglyceride level and hypercholesterolemia</li><li>Age: men over 40 years and women over 50 years</li><li>Symptoms lasting for 30–60 minutes</li></ul> |
| Pericarditis | <ul><li>Sharp or stabbing chest pain over the centre or left side of the chest</li><li>Increased pain with deep breathing, swallowing, coughing or left-side lying</li><li>Relieved with forward leaning and sitting up</li><li>Shortness of breath, heart palpitations, fatigue, nausea</li></ul> |

| Condition | Signs and symptoms |
|---|---|
| Pneumothorax | • Intensified pain the chest during inspiration, ventilation or expanding of rib cage<br>• Abnormally rapid breathing<br>• Hypotension, dyspnea or hypoxia<br>• Distant or absent sounds of breath |
| Pneumonia | • Sharp and piercing chest pain while breathing or coughing<br>• Fever, shaking chills, headache, sweating, fatigue or nausea<br>• Productive cough |
| Fracture | • Greater than 70 years of age<br>• Recent history of major trauma<br>• Prolonged use of corticosteroids<br>• History of osteoporosis |
| Tumour | • History of cancer (e.g. breast carcinoma and lung carcinoma)<br>• Suspected malignancy<br>• Unexplained deformity, mass or swelling |
| Infection, septic arthritis | • Red skin<br>• Systemically unwell such as loss of appetite or unusual fatigue (malaise)<br>• Constitutional symptoms such as recent fever, chills or unexplained weight loss<br>• Recent bacterial infection<br>• Severe and/or persisting shoulder complaints |

Sources: Mitchell *et al.* (2005); Mutsaers and van Dolder (2008); Dutton (2012); Magee (2014)

## Special Tests

### Table 13.5 Special tests for measuring serious pathology in the shoulder and rib cage

| Test | Procedure | Positive sign | Interpretation |
|---|---|---|---|
| Hawkins' impingement test | The examiner forward flexes the patient's arm and elbow to 90°. The examiner then applies a force to the arm to internally rotate the shoulder at the glenohumeral joint. | • Pain on internal rotation | ☐ Subacromial impingement or rotator cuff tendonitis |

| | | | |
|---|---|---|---|
| Drop-arm rotator cuff test | The examiner passively abducts the patient's arm to 160°. The patient is then instructed to slowly lower the arm to the waist. | • Inability to control the manoeuvre as far as the side | ☐ Supraspinatus or rotator cuff tear |
| Apprehension test | The patient is placed in either supine lying or sitting position. The examiner applies anterior pressure on the humerus while externally rotating the patient's arm. | • Sensation of apprehension or resistance | ☐ Glenohumeral instability |
| Empty-can test | The examiner abducts the patient's arms to 90° and then forward flexes to 30°. With the patient's thumbs turned downward, the examiner applies pressure. The patient actively resists to the downward force. | • Pain or weakness compared with the contralateral side | ☐ Supraspinatus tendon or muscle tear |
| Anterior-posterior rib compression test | For this manoeuvre, the patient can be in either sitting or standing position. The examiner stands laterally to the patient and places one hand on the anterior and another on the posterior aspects of the rib cage. The examiner compresses the rib cage by pushing the hands together and then releases the pressure. | • The rib shaft being prominent in the midaxillary line<br>• Pain or point tenderness with the rib-cage compression<br>• Respiratory restrictions for both inhalation and exhalation | ☐ Possibly a rib fracture, contusion or separation |

| Test | Procedure | Positive sign | Interpretation |
|---|---|---|---|
| Chest expansion test | With the patient in either seated or standing position, the examiner places his/her thumbs near to the patient's 10th ribs. The fingers of the examiner are in parallel to the lateral rib cage, loosely grasping the lower hemithorax on either side of axilla. The examiner then slides his/her hands medially just sufficient to elevate a loose skin fold between the thumbs. The patient is asked to breathe and expire deeply.<br><br>Next, the examiner stands in front of the patient and places his/her thumbs laterally to each costal margin, with the hands along the lateral rib cage. The examiner then slides his/her hands medially to elevate a loose skin fold between the thumbs. The patient is asked to breathe and expire deeply. The examiner notes the space between the thumbs in both posterior and anterior aspects and feels for the symmetry of movement of the hemithorax. | • Asymmetrical chest expansion<br>• Abnormal side expands less and lags behind the normal side | ☐ Unilateral decrease or delay in chest expansion indicates pathology on that side, such as lobar pneumonia, pleural effusion and unilateral bronchial obstruction<br>☐ Bilateral decrease in chest expansion is usually suggests chronic obstructive pulmonary disease (COPD) or asthma |

| Rib-cage respiratory test | **Ribs 1–10:** The patient lies in supine position. The therapist palpates directly over the ribs anteriorly, particularly on the intercostal spaces. The patient is then asked to make a full inspiratory and expiratory effort. The therapist should then assess the respiratory excursion for the superior and inferior ribs. | • One group of ribs stops moving first during either inhalation or exhalation | ☐ Rib dysfunction |
| | **Ribs 11 and 12:** The patient lies in prone position. The therapist's hand is symmetrically placed over the 11th and 12th ribs posteriorly. The patient is once again asked to make a full inspiratory and expiratory effort. The therapist should then palpate the movement and assess the respiratory excursion. | | |

Sources: Magee (2014); Burbank *et al.* (2008); Woodward and Best (2000); Bickley and Szilagyi (2012); Bookhout (1996); Tuteur (1990)

# References

Bickley, L. and Szilagyi, P.G. (2012). *Bates' Guide to Physical Examination and History-Taking*. Philadelphia, PA: Lippincott Williams & Wilkins.

Bigliani, L.U., Kelkar, R., Flatow, E.L., Pollock, R.G. and Mow, V.C. (1996). Glenohumeral Stability: Biomechanical properties of passive and active stabilizers. *Clinical Orthopaedics and Related Research, 330*, 13–30.

Bontrager, K.L. and Lampignano, J. (2013). *Textbook of Radiographic Positioning and Related Anatomy*. St Louis, MO: Elsevier Health Sciences.

Bookhout, R.M. (1996). Evaluation of the thoracic spine and rib cage. In T.W. Flynn (Ed.), *The Thoracic Spine and Rib Cage*. Oxford: Butterworth-Heinemann Medical.

Burbank, K.M., Stevenson, J.H., Czarnecki, G.R. and Dorfman, J. (2008). Chronic shoulder pain: Part I. Evaluation and diagnosis. *American Family Physician, 77*(4), 453–460.

Crooper, R.J. (1996). Regional anatomy and biomechanics. In T.W. Flynn (Ed.), *The Thoracic Spine and Rib Cage*. Butterworth-Heinemann Medical.

Dala-Ali, B., Penna, M., McConnell, J., Vanhegan, I. and Cobiella, C. (2012). Management of acute anterior shoulder dislocation. *British Journal of Sports Medicine, 48*(16), 1209–1215.

Duprey, S., Subit, D., Guillemot, H. and Kent, R.W. (2010). Biomechanical properties of the costovertebral joint. *Medical Engineering and Physics, 32*(2), 222–227.

Dutton, M. (2012). *Dutton's Orthopaedic Examination Evaluation and Intervention*. New York, NY: McGraw-Hill Professional.

Ekholm, R., Adami, J., Tidermark, J., Hansson, K., Törnkvist, H. and Ponzer, S. (2006). Fractures of the shaft of the humerus an epidemiological study of 401 fractures. *Journal of Bone and Joint Surgery, 88*(11), 1469–1473.

Ernst, E. (2007). Adverse effects of spinal manipulation: A systematic review. *Journal of the Royal Society of Medicine, 100*(7), 330–338.

Halder, A.M., Itoi, E. and An, K.N. (2000). Anatomy and biomechanics of the shoulder. *Orthopedic Clinics of North America, 31*(2), 159–176.

Jeray, K.J. (2007). Acute midshaft clavicular fracture. *Journal of the American Academy of Orthopaedic Surgeons, 15*(4), 239–248.

Khan, L.K., Bradnock, T.J., Scott, C. and Robinson, C.M, (2009). Fractures of the clavicle. *The Journal of Bone and Joint Surgery, 91*(2), 447–460.

Krøner, K., Lind, T. and Jensen, J. (1989). The epidemiology of shoulder dislocations. *Archives of Orthopaedic and Trauma Surgery, 108*(5), 288–290.

Lason, G. and Peeters, L. (2014). The shoulder (Vol. 2). *The Shoulder, the Elbow, the Wrist and the Hand*. The International Academy of Osteopathy.

Liman, S.T., Kuzucu, A., Tastepe, A.I., Ulasan, G.N. and Topcu, S. (2003). Chest injury due to blunt trauma. *European Journal of Cardio-Thoracic Surgery, 23*(3), 374–378.

Lynch, T.S., Saltzman, M.D., Ghodasra, J.H., Bilimoria, K.Y., Bowen, M.K. and Nuber, G.W. (2013). Acromioclavicular joint injuries in the National Football League: Epidemiology and management. *American Journal of Sports Medicine, 41*(12), 2904–2908.

Mader, S.S. (2004). *Understanding Human Anatomy and Physiology*. McGraw-Hill Science.

Magee, D.J. (2014). *Orthopedic Physical Assessment*. Elsevier Health Sciences.

Melendez, L.S. and Doty, I.C. (2015). Rib fractures. *eMedicine*. Available at http://emedicine. medscape.com/article/825981-overview#showall (accessed 30 July 2016).

Mitchell, C., Adebajo, A., Hay, E. and Carr, A. (2005). Shoulder pain: Diagnosis and management in primary care. *British Medical Journal, 331*(7525), 1124–1128.

Moses, S. (2007). Shoulder range of motion. *Family Practice Notebook*. Available at www. fpnotebook.com/ortho/exam/shldrrngofmtn.htm (accessed 30 July 2016).

Mutsaers, B. and van Dolder, R. (2008). *'Red Flags' of the Neck and Shoulder Area: A Review of the Literature*. Available at http://vanpend.nl/Publicatie20_DTO_PDF.pdf (accessed 30 July 2016).

Ombregt, L. (2003). The thoracic spine: Disorders of the thoracic cage and abdomen. In L. Ombregt, P. Bisschop and H.J. ter Veer (Eds), *A System of Orthopaedic Medicine*, 2nd edition. Churchill Livingstone.

Palastanga, N. and Soames, R. (2011). *Anatomy and Human Movement*, 6th edition. Elsevier Health Sciences.

Quillen, D.M., Wuchner, M. and Hatch, R.L. (2004). Acute shoulder injuries. *American Family Physician, 70*(10), 1947–1954.

Rivett, D.A., Thomas, L. and Bolton, B. (2005). Premanipulative testing: Where do we go from here? *New Zealand Journal of Physiotherapy, 33*(3), 78–84.

Rockwood Jr, C.A., Matsen III, F.A., Wirth, M.A. and Lippitt, S.B. (2009). *The Shoulder*. Elsevier Health Sciences.

Sofu, H., Gürsu, S., Koçkara, N., Öner, A., Issın, A. and Çamurcu, Y. (2014). Recurrent anterior shoulder instability: Review of the literature and current concepts. *World Journal of Clinical Cases, 2*(11), 676.

Terry, G.C. and Chopp, T.M. (2000). Functional anatomy of the shoulder. *Journal of Athletic Training, 35*(3), 248–255.

Tuteur, P.G. (1990). Chest examination. In H.K. Walker, W.D. Hall and J.W. Hurst (Eds), *Clinical Methods: The History, Physical, and Laboratory Examinations*. Butterworths. Available at www.ncbi.nlm.nih.gov/books/NBK368 (accessed 30 July 2016).

Van Tongel, A., MacDonald, P., Leiter, J., Pouliart, N. and Peeler, J. (2012). A cadaveric study of the structural anatomy of the sternoclavicular joint. *Clinical Anatomy, 25*(7), 903–910.

White, T.D. and Folkens, P.A. (2005). *The Human Bone Manual*. Academic Press.

William, E., Glynn, E.P. and Cleland, J.A. (2015). Thoracic spine manipulation. In: *Manual therapy for musculoskeletal pain syndromes: An Evidence- and Clinical-Informed Approach*. Churchill Livingstone.

Woodward, T.W. and Best, T.M. (2000). The painful shoulder: Part I. Clinical evaluation. *American Family Physician, 61*(10), 3079–3089.

World Health Organization (2005). *WHO Guidelines on Basic Training and Safety in Chiropractic*. Geneva: World Health Organization.

Yoganandan, N. and Pintar, F.A. (1998). Biomechanics of human thoracic ribs. *Journal of Biomechanical Engineering, 120*(1), 100–104.

Zlowodzki, M., Zelle, B.A., Cole, P.A., Jeray, K. and McKee, M.D. (2005). Treatment of acute midshaft clavicle fractures: Systematic review of 2144 fractures: on behalf of the Evidence-Based Orthopaedic Trauma Working Group. *Journal of Orthopaedic Trauma, 19*(7), 504–507.

# Techniques for the Shoulder and Rib Cage

## Prone Contralateral Rib

- This technique is applicable for R2–R5.
- Stand facing the patient.
- Locate the rib angle or costotransverse joint of the target segment.
- Using the lower hand, apply a pisiform contact over the target segment.
- Remove skin slack by sliding the skin, muscle and fascia accordingly.
- Using your support hand, compress the contact hand with elbows locked.
- Ask the patient to breathe deeply in, then out, following the rib as it drops away from your hand.
- At the end of the exhalation, apply a manipulation through your legs directly PA towards the table.

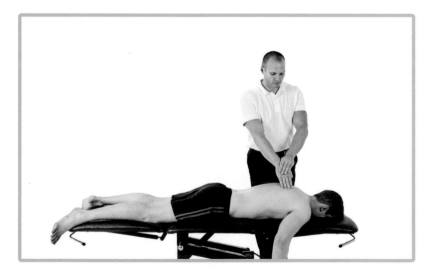

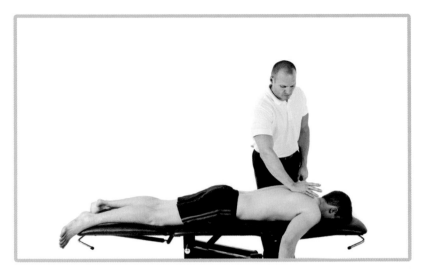

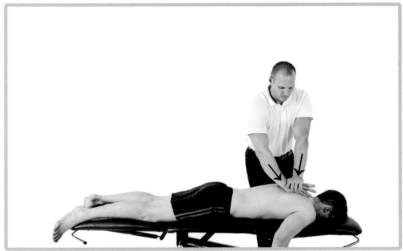

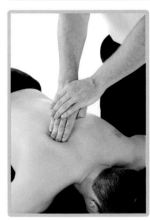
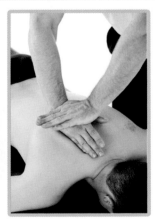

**Key Points**

- Locating a rib is best done with the patient's arms dropped off the side of the table.
- Patient breathing and skin slack are vital for localising movement and maintaining your contact.
- Be sure to lock your arms to enable an effective body drop thrust.
- Do not recoil before administering your manipulation; it should be a continuation of the tension created by expiration and a posterior to anterior pressure.
- Do not use excessive pressure during the loading or tension phase; this can cause pain and reflex muscle spasm.

# Prone Rib Technique

- This technique is suitable for ribs 3–10.
- Stand facing the patient.
- Use an asymmetrical stance with the same leg in front as the hand holding the ASIS (i.e. right arm and right leg).
- Contact the patient's ASIS.
- With your superior hand, contact the chosen rib angle.
- Ask the patient to breathe deeply in, then out.
- As the patient is halfway through the breath-out phase, rotate the trunk by pulling the ASIS towards you while you apply a downward pressure to the rib angle until you feel the barrier.
- Simultaneously thrust directly towards the table with your superior hand and pull anterior to posterior with the inferior hand to apply the manipulation.

**Key Points**

- Your front leg should be in contact with the table to aid leverage.
- Be patient with this technique as it is all about working with the rhythm of the patient's breathing.
- Use your body to gain power during this technique. Rotate towards the superior leg with the rib contact arm locked in place with full elbow extension.

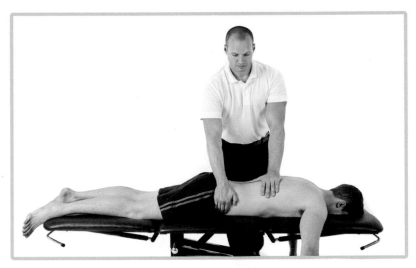

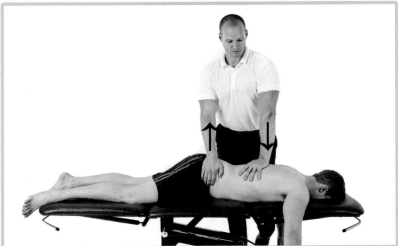

- Use your legs to body drop into a lunge to create the posterior to anterior thrust on the rib.
- The higher up the body the rib, the more muscular, joint and fascial slack will need to be taken with your inferior ASIS contact.

## Supine Rib Contralateral Contact

- This technique is applicable between R2 and R10.
- The patient is in supine position.
- Stand at the side of the patient in an asymmetrical stance with the outermost leg forward.

215

TECHNIQUE

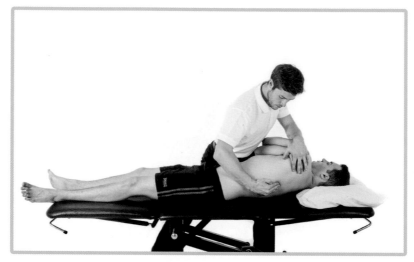

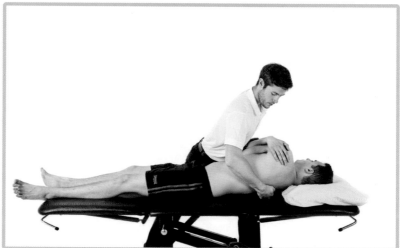

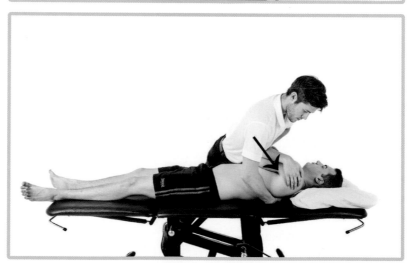

- Ask the patient to cross their arms one on top of the other in a V shape.
- Reach to the patient's opposite shoulder with your left hand ideally contacting the medial border of the scapula.
- Roll the patient towards you, revealing the contralateral rib angles.
- Locate the desired rib and create a thenar contact or fist contact with your right hand.
- Do not roll the patient back over just yet. Ask them to inhale.
- Halfway through the exhalation, roll the patient back on to your right hand. The dorsal aspect of your right hand should make contact with the table.
- Using your left hand, move the patient's elbows above where your right hand is in contact with the rib you want to manipulate.
- As the pressure on your contact hand begins to build up, you will have reached the barrier, so with a drop through your legs perform the manipulation.

**Key Points**
- Locating rib angles is done best by crossing the patient's arms to remove the overlying scapula.
- Patient breathing and skin slack are vital for localising movement and maintaining your contact.
- Your body and hand contact of the patient's elbow needs to be firmly locked in position to ensure the transfer of movement into the patient's rib angle.
- Do not roll on to the contact point too early as the high level of pressure can cause reflex spasm and pain, making it hard to effectively manipulate the area.
- Maintain a straight back posture, using your hips to move both you and the patient.

## Rolling Rib Manipulation – Ipsilateral Contact

- This technique is applicable for R2–R10.
- Assist the patient to a seated position.
- Direct the patient to raise the contralateral knee into a relaxed flexion position.

TECHNIQUE

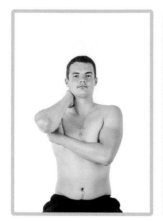

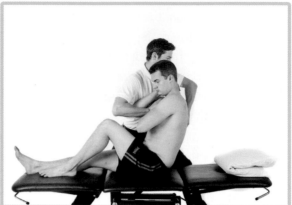

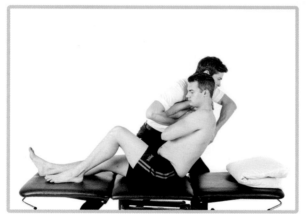

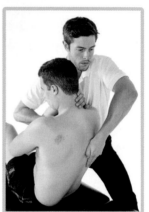

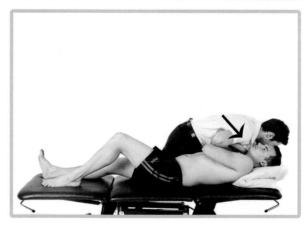

- Ask the patient to raise the ipsilateral arm to hold behind the neck, their elbow facing directly upward.
- The patient's opposite hand should then be placed underneath this arm with their hand directly covering the axilla.
- Lunge with your left leg forward.
- With your left hand, reach over the patient's ipsilateral shoulder to find your contact on the desired rib angle.
- Use a thenar contact with fingers pointing directly inferior.
- With the opposite support hand, cover the patient's hand overlying the axilla area.
- With the medial aspect of the same arm, pull their raised elbow into your body; this will enable you to control their upper body and create tension.
- Ask them to drop their head and slump as if to relax.
- Direct the patient to inhale and exhale.
- As they exhale, roll the patient down on to your contact hand while keeping your body in contact with the patient's.
- Using the patient's raised elbow and lunging through your legs, engage the barrier through the patient's elbow and shoulder to pressure enabling tension to build over the rib contact hand underneath.
- Manipulate via lunging through your legs, AP to the table.

**Key Points**
- Locating a rib is best done with the arm raised as it clears the scapula away from the rib cage.
- The contact arm is raised to keep the therapist's forearm away from contacting the scapula and blocking the ribs' movement.
- Patient breathing and skin slack are vital for localising movement and maintaining your contact.
- Be sure to lock your body and the patient's arm and shoulder together to ensure the correct transfer of force and ability to locate tension.
- Do not recoil before administering your thrust; it should be a continuation of the tension created by expiration and anterior to posterior, inferior to superior pressure.
- Do not use excessive pressure during the loading or tension phase; this can cause pain and reflex muscle spasm.
- Raising the leg will relax those with lower back pain.

### Alternative

- This technique can be completed with the patient supine and your contact arm reversed with radial border of your contact hand along the medial border of the scapula. The technique remains the same as above.

## Seated Rotational Rib Manipulation

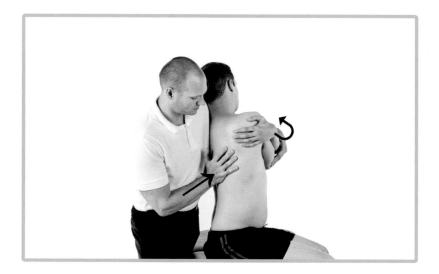

- This technique is applicable for R3–R10.
- Stand behind the seated patient.
- Ask the patient to cross their arms one on top of the other.
- Reach around the patient to contact the inferior elbow.
- Rotate yourself so that your supporting shoulder is contacting the patient.
- With your free hand, locate the selected rib angle.
- Using a pisiform contact, take out any skin slack to prevent slipping.
- Drop your elbow downward to enable an inferior to superior line of drive.
- Ask the patient to inhale and exhale.
- Take the patient to the barrier by rotating them away from the side of contact aided by your support hand.
- When the barrier is engaged, manipulate obliquely through the rib angle while rotating the patient away from the involved segment.

**Key Points**

- Locating rib angles is best done by crossing the patient's arms to remove the overlying scapula.
- Patient breathing and skin slack are vital for localising movement and maintaining your contact.
- Your body and hand contact of the patient's elbow need to be firmly locked in position to ensure the transfer of movement into the patient's rib angle.
- Move the patient towards the back of the bench to limit the amount of reaching involved.
- Use your legs and body to thrust, rather than your arms, to create more power while protecting your body.
- Do not perform this technique if the patient has a known lumbar spine dysfunction as the rotation may aggravate this.

# Seated R1 Technique

- This technique is applicable for R1.
- Stand behind the patient.
- Raise your contralateral leg on to the bench.
- Take the patient's arm and lay it over your raised thigh.
- Ask the patient to rest their opposite arm on their thigh.
- With your supporting hand, contact the patient's contralateral temporal region.
- Locate the R1.
- With your thumb and first finger, contact R1.
- Laterally shift the patient by drawing them towards your raised leg.
- As soft-tissue resistance is reached, engage the barrier by applying pressure from SI with your contact hand.

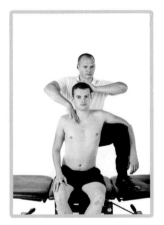

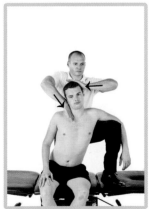

- At the same time apply an opposing force to side-bend the head (via a temporal contact with your palm) to engage the barrier.
- Ask the patient to breathe deeply in, then out.
- Simultaneously manipulate SI to LM, towards the axilla with your contact hand and LM with your support hand.

**Key Points**
- Locating the first rib is best done by palpating just posterior to the clavicle.
- Patient breathing and skin slack are vital for localising movement and maintaining your contact.
- Move the patient to the back of the bench to reduce the amount of reaching involved.
- Gain consent before applying the arm contact.

# Ipsilateral Prone R1 Technique

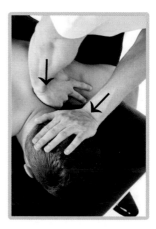

- Stand on the side of the table with an asymmetrical stance.
- Your right hand palpates and contacts R1 via your pisiform. Lock out your right elbow and slightly internally rotate your right shoulder.
- Your left hand contacts the side of the head via the temporal bone just above the ear.
- Ask the patient to inhale and exhale.
- Halfway through the exhalation phase, add PA compression with your right hand to engage the barrier, at the same time rotating the head with your left hand.
- Your left arm should be parallel to the table.
- Once the barrier is engaged, manipulate R1 with a PA movement through your right hand and rotation of the cervical spine with your left.

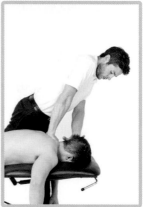

**Key Points**

- Keep your left arm parallel to the table and do not raise it too high; otherwise, you will push the patient's face into the face hole.
- Make sure you wait for the patient to exhale fully.
- When manipulating R1, do not forget to use your legs and not your arm strength.

# Glenohumeral Manipulation

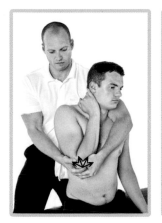 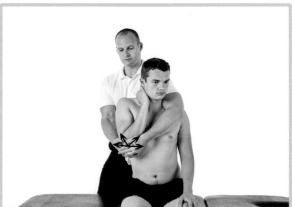

- This technique is performed seated.
- Ask the patient to place the palmar surface of their hand (on the side to be manipulated) on the posterior surface of their neck.
- Stand behind the patient with an asymmetrical stance.
- Use a towel to help make a stable contact with the patient and do not block the movement of the scapula.
- Secure your hands around the olecranon of the elbow by interlocking your fingers.
- Ask the patient to inhale and exhale.
- At the end of the exhalation phase, the barrier should be engaged.
- The manipulation is performed AP.
- You can change the angle of the manipulation to suit the needs of the patient.

### Key Points

- Make sure the patient is not slouching prior to starting and that their head is in a neutral position.
- Make sure the arm on the contralateral side to be manipulated is not compressing the side of the patient's neck.
- This technique can also be used for the acromioclavicular joint by using the towel to help block the scapula movement. This helps focus the manipulation more to this joint.
- Do not perform this manipulation if this is any caution relating to shoulder stability or elbow pathology.
- This technique can help gain mobility for patients with adhesive capsulitis.

## Shoulder Humeral Head Manipulation

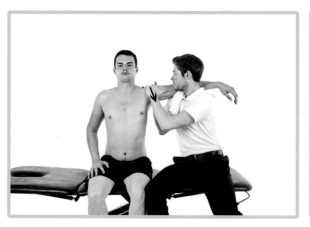 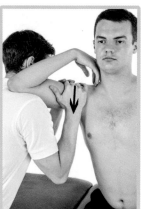

- The patient is seated or recumbent.
- Sit or stand next to the patient, facing them on the side to be manipulated.
- The patient's arm is extended and their cubital fossa supported by the practitioner's shoulder.
- The practitioner's fingers are interlinked, spanning across the anterior surface of the proximal humerus with palms supporting the medial and lateral aspects.
- The patient is asked to inhale and exhale.

- To engage the barrier, compress your hands slightly securing your grip over the humerus and manipulate inferior.

**Key Points**
- You do not need to use force at all with this technique.
- Proceed with caution with patients with glenohumeral stability problems.
- This technique can be performed with the patient's elbow flexed if preferred.
- You can place a towel over your shoulder and clavicle to avoid discomfort on the patient's arm.
- Your interlinked hands should be covering the proximal humeral head along the AC joint line and not over the AC joint.

## Seated Acromioclavicular Manipulation

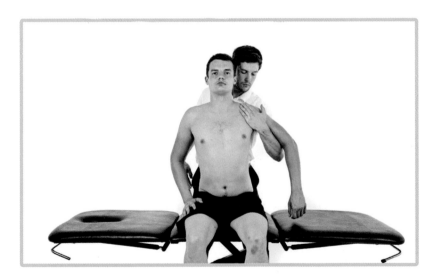

- The patient is seated.
- Stand behind the patient and use a towel on their thoracic SPs to gain a secure contact with the patient.
- Place your left hand on the anterior aspect of the AC joint.
- The palmar aspect can then be placed on the anterior of the glenohumeral with the second metacarpal resting over the mid portion of the anterior clavicle.

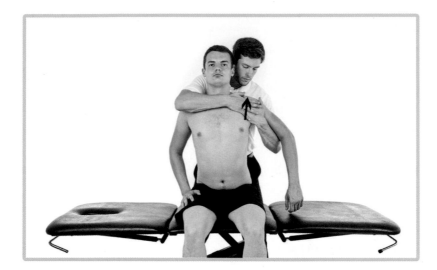

- Your secondary hand is then used to reinforce the applicator by placing the forearm across the patient's upper torso.
- The patient is asked to inhale and exhale.
- At the end of the exhalation phase, engage the barrier by moving the AC joint posterior superior (PS) and adding compression posterior.
- Perform the manipulation.

### Key Points
- Do not perform this technique on patients after AC ligament repair or replacement.
- Be cautious on patients who have history of clavicle fractures.

## Sternoclavicular Manipulation

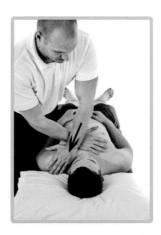

- The patient is in supine position.
- Stand to the side of plinth of the SC joint to be manipulated, facing towards the patient with an asymmetrical stance.
- Your left pisiform fixes on to the medial head of the clavicle and your left on to the sternum.
- The patient is asked inhale and exhale.

- At the very end of exhalation. the barrier is engaged by adding lateral compression to the clavicle and lateral compression to the sternum.
- Perform the manipulation once barrier is engaged.

**Key Points**

- Contact the sternum and makes sure you are below the sternal notch and point your fingers away from the patient's throat.
- The time between barrier engagement and manipulation is very small.
- Be careful not to compress the distal attachment of the sterno-cleidomastoid and scalene muscles as this will likely cause pain – fix only on the anterior surface of the clavicle.

# CHAPTER 14

# The Elbow, Wrist and Hand

## Introduction

Over the last century, the use of thrust manipulation to treat upper extremity pathologies has increased progressively. Today manipulation is now used as an adjunctive therapy for a range of upper limb disorders, including lateral epicondylitis, nursemaid's elbow, post-traumatic elbow stiffness, carpal tunnel syndrome, cubital tunnel syndrome and many more (Lason and Peeters, 2014). Advocates of manual therapy consider manipulation a relatively safe and effective approach to treat upper extremity disorders. In addition, they claim that a great majority of patients with musculoskeletal pathologies can benefit from manipulative procedures (Paterson and Burn, 2012).

Practitioners of manipulative therapy use various techniques depending on the upper extremity joint and/or lesion being treated. The therapeutic goal of these practitioners is to apply a procedure that is well tolerated by the recipient and yields the best result. They primarily aim to reduce inflammation, alleviate spasticity, correct malalignment of bones, decrease overload of forces, promote faster healing and increase upper extremity strength, endurance and flexibility (Saunders et al., 2015). In general, they usually utilise two manipulation approaches for manual correction of upper extremity abnormalities: high-velocity, low-amplitude thrust (HVLAT) and mobilisation.

However, despite many positive claims by the advocates of manual therapy, there has been a lack of quality research and evidence in support of manipulation of the upper extremity (Bronfort *et al.*, 2010). Given the limited evidence with regard to the therapy, the benefits and risks associated with upper extremity manipulation are yet not explored (Brantingham *et al.*, 2013; McHardy *et al.*, 2008). Therefore, before deciding to perform a manipulative procedure, a practitioner must make sure that no absolute contraindication or red flag for serious pathology is present. Moreover, because adequate knowledge, good technical skill, extensive experience and sound clinical reasoning play an important role in preventing incidence of adverse events following manipulation, it is of critical importance for practitioners to have appropriate training and education (World Health Organization, 2005; Ernst, 2007; Brantingham *et al.*, 2013).

The purpose of this chapter is to help practitioners diagnose serious pathologies of the upper extremity. However, as we have already discussed the shoulder region in a separate chapter, this chapter will particularly focus on the elbow, wrist and hand. In addition, this chapter will also describe the various joints of these structures, the range of motion in these joints, some common injuries to the regions and the red flags for manipulation.

## Joints

In human anatomy, the upper extremity is the region that extends from the deltoid region to the hand. It includes all the structures from the shoulder to the hand. The elbow acts as a mechanical link between the shoulder and the hand. The major functions of the elbow comprise placing the hand in space, serving as a hinge or support for the forearm and affording fine movements of the hand and wrist (Alcid, Ahmad and Lee, 2004).

In contrast, the hand and wrist comprise a complex system of static and dynamic structures, consisting of bones, muscles, tendons, ligaments and skin. Together they perform a variety of complex tasks, including object handling, providing oppositional grip, communicating and various other tasks in daily life (Doyle, 2003).

**Table 14.1 The joints of the elbow, wrist and hand**

| Joint name | Description | Function |
|---|---|---|
| Elbow joint | • A highly congruous and stable joint<br>• Forms a complex hinge between three bones: the humerus, the ulna and the radius<br>• Involves three separate articulations: the humeroulnar joint, the humeroradial joint and the superior radioulnar joint<br>• Surrounded by a single fibrous capsule that encloses the entire joint complex | • Provides the arm with much of its versatility and allows the hand to move towards and away from the body<br>• Allows flexion and extension of the upper arm as well as supination and pronation of the forearm and wrist |
| Humeroulnar joint | • A synovial hinge joint, which is one of the three joints that constitute the elbow<br>• Composed of two bones: the humerus and the ulna<br>• Originates from the trochlear notch of the ulna to the trochlear of the humeral condyle<br>• Involves articulation between the humerus and the ulna | • Allows flexion and extension of the elbow |
| Humeroradial joint | • A ball-and-socket joint, which is one of the three joints that constitute the elbow<br>• Originates from the superior aspect of the radial head to the capitulum of the humeral condyle<br>• Involves articulation between the humerus and the radius | • Allows flexion and extension of the elbow with rotation of the radial head on the capitellum |

| Superior radioulnar joint | • A pivot-type synovial joint that is encapsulated within the elbow's synovial tissue<br>• Originates from the head of the radius to the radial notch of the ulna | • Allows pronation or supination movement of the elbow |
|---|---|---|
| Radiocarpal joint | • A major synovial joint formed between the forearm and the hand<br>• Connects the distal radius to the scaphoid, lunate and triquetrum | • Contributes to the stability of the wrist<br>• Allows the wrist to move along two axes<br>• Supports flexion, extension, adduction and abduction of the wrist |
| Intercarpal joints | • Synovial joints that involve articulations between the individual carpal bones of the wrist<br>• Subdivided into three sets of articulations: joints of the proximal row, joints of the distal row and joints between these two rows | • Contribute to total wrist mobility |
| Midcarpal joint | • A synovial, S-shaped joint formed between the proximal and distal carpal rows<br>• Composed of a very extensive and irregular joint cavity | • Allows the initial phase of wrist flexion and extension |
| Carpometacarpal joints | • Synovial joints formed between the distal row of carpal bones and the proximal row of metacarpal bones<br>• Supported by some strong ligaments, including the carpometacarpal and pisometacarpal ligaments | • Contribute to the palmar arch system in the hand |
| Intermetacarpal joints | • Plane synovial joints formed between the metacarpals<br>• Occur between the bases of the second, third, fourth and fifth metacarpal bones<br>• Strengthened by a group of ligaments, including the dorsal, palmar and interosseous metacarpal ligaments | • Permit some flexion-extension and adjunct rotation |

| Joint name | Description | Function |
|---|---|---|
| Metacarpophalangeal joints | • Condyloid-type joints that connect the distal head of metacarpals to the proximal phalanges of the fingers<br>• Supported by a number of ligaments, including the strong palmar and collateral ligaments | • Allow movement of the fingers in different directions (e.g. flexion, extension, abduction, adduction and circumduction) |
| Interphalangeal joints | • Hinge joints formed between the phalanges of the fingers<br>• Connect the heads of the phalanges to the bases of the next distal phalanges<br>• Subdivided into two sets of articulations: proximal interphalangeal joints and distal interphalangeal joints | • Allow flexion and extension movements |

Sources: Alcid *et al.* (2004); Kuxhaus (2008); Fornalski, Gupta and Lee (2003); McCann and Wise (2011); Standring (2008); Doyle (2003)

## Range of Motion

The elbow joint is a complex hinge between three bones and thus involves three separate articulations: the humeroulnar joint, the humeroradial joint and the radioulnar joint. These three joints comprise a single compound joint and work in coordination to allow flexion and extension of the upper arm and, at the same time, supination and pronation of the forearm and wrist (Villaseñor-Ovies *et al.*, 2012).

**Table 14.2 Normal range of motion of the elbow joint**

| Movement type | Range of motion |
|---|---|
| Flexion | 140–150° |
| Extension | 0° |
| Pronation | 76–84° |
| Supination | 80° |

Source: Norkin and White (2009)

## Table 14.3 Range of motion of elbow for activities of daily living

| Movement type | Range of motion |
|---|---|
| Flexion | 75–120° |
| Extension | 0° |
| Pronation | 50° |
| Supination | 50° |

Sources: Vasen *et al.* (1995); Morrey, Askew and Chao (1981)

In contrast to the elbow joint, the hand and wrist have an incredible range of motion and help assist in a wide range of activities of daily living.

## Table 14.4 Normal range of motion of the wrist

| Movement type | Range of motion |
|---|---|
| Flexion | 60–80° |
| Extension | 60 75° |
| Radial deviation | 20–25° |
| Ulnar deviation | 30–39° |

Source: Norkin and White (2009)

## Table 14.5 Functional and average range of motion of the wrist

| Motion unit | Range of motion | Reference |
|---|---|---|
| Functional range of motion in ADL | • 45° of flexion<br>• 50° of extension<br>• 15° of radial deviation<br>• 40° of ulnar deviation | Brigstocke *et al.* (2013) |
| Average range of motion in ADL | • 50° of flexion<br>• 51° of extension<br>• 12° of radial deviation<br>• 40° of ulnar deviation | Nelson *et al.* (1994) |

**Table 14.6 Normal range of motion of the finger joints**

| Joint name | Motion type | Average |
|---|---|---|
| Metacarpophalangeal joint | Flexion | 90–100° |
| | Extension | 20–45° |
| Proximal interphalangeal joint | Flexion | 90–120° |
| | Extension | 0° |
| Distal interphalangeal joint | Flexion | 70–90° |
| | Extension | 0° |
| Metacarpophalangeal joint (thumb) | Flexion | 50–60° |
| | Extension | 14–23° |
| Interphalangeal joint (thumb) | Flexion | 67–80° |
| Carpometacarpal joint (thumb) | Flexion | 15–45° |
| | Extension | 0–20° |
| | Abduction | 50–70° |

Sources: Norkin and White (2009); Floyd and Thompson (2004)

## Common Injuries

A major injury to the elbow, wrist and hand is often caused by a fall, motor vehicle accident, violent activity, sport accident or penetrating trauma. These injuries can result in significant disability and upset activities of daily living. In addition, they are common in all populations, including male and female, the very young and the old, and participants of numerous sports.

Elbow injuries are more common in athletes of all ages and skill levels, especially in sports involving overhead arm motions (e.g. throwing and racquet sports) (Whiteside, Andrews and Fleisig, 1999). However, the wrist and hand are the most injured parts of the body. While the fingers account for 38.4% of all injuries, the wrist accounts for 15.2% of all upper extremity injuries (Ootes, Lambers and Ring, 2012).

## Table 14.7 Common injuries to the elbow, wrist and hand

| Common injuries | Characteristics |
| --- | --- |
| Dislocation of the radial head or pulled elbow | <ul><li>Often comes with significant trauma</li><li>Occurs when the radial head is pulled out of the anular ligament</li><li>Results in displacement of the radial head from its normal articulation with the humerus and the ulna</li><li>In children, the head of the radius is more frequently subluxed than dislocated</li><li>Occurs most commonly in male adults who are subject to high-force injury</li><li>Peak incidence occurs in young children (under the age of 5), more frequently in girls</li></ul> |
| Lateral epicondylitis | <ul><li>A condition in which the lateral epicondyle of the humerus becomes sore and tender</li><li>Involves an acute or chronic inflammation and micro-tearing of fibres in the extensor tendons</li><li>Results from overuse of the wrist extensor musculature, such as extensor carpi radialis brevis</li><li>Occurs in more than 50% of athletes who use overhead arm motions</li><li>Annual incidence: 4–7 cases per 1000 patients</li><li>Peak incidence: 40–50 years of age</li></ul> |
| Olecranon bursitis | <ul><li>An inflammation of the olecranon bursa, which is located just above the extensor aspect of the ulna's proximal end</li><li>Characterised by pain, swelling and redness near the olecranon process</li><li>Often occurs due to prolonged pressure, single injury to the elbow, mild but repeated minor injuries, infection, trauma or other condition that aggravate inflammation</li><li>Pick incidence occurs at older age</li></ul> |
| Wrist bone fracture (scaphoid) | <ul><li>A common bone fracture in the carpus region</li><li>May involve direct axial compression or hyperextension of the wrist</li><li>Occurs more often in men than in women</li><li>Most common in young men (age group: 15–29 years) following a fall, athletic injury or motor vehicle accident on an outstretched hand</li><li>Symptoms include pain in wrist motion, swelling around the wrist and tenderness in wrist and at the thumb base</li></ul> |

| Mallet finger | • An injury of the extensor digitorum tendon of the fingers<br>• Results from interruption of the terminal extensor mechanism at the distal interphalangeal joint<br>• Usually occurs when an object strikes the finger and creates a forceful flexion of an extended distal interphalangeal joint<br>• Symptoms include tenderness just behind nail, pain and swelling at the end of the injured finger, and inability to straighten the tip of that finger |
|---|---|
| De Quervain syndrome | • A tenosynovitis of the sheath that involves the abductor pollicis longus and the extensor pollicis brevis<br>• Usually develops due to a direct blow to the wrist, thumb or tendon, repetitive grasping, overuse of the wrist and certain inflammatory conditions<br>• Occurs most commonly in the middle-aged<br>• Affects women 8–10 times more often than men<br>• Symptoms include difficulty gripping, pain and tenderness on certain movements of the wrist, and pain along the base of the thumb |
| Carpal tunnel syndrome | • A condition in which the median nerve is compressed as it traverses the tunnel under the thick transverse carpal ligament<br>• Often develops due to forceful or repetitive hand and wrist movements, which in turn irritate or compress the median nerve in the wrist<br>• Usually occurs in middle-aged (age group: 30–60 years), obese women<br>• Prevalence is almost four times more often in older women than in men<br>• May be associated with myxoedema, acromegaly, pregnancy, obesity, rheumatoid arthritis, primary amyloidosis, tophaceous gout and repetitive work with the hand<br>• Symptoms include numbness, tingling, pain and weakness in the palm of the hand and the fingers |

Sources: Ovesen *et al.* (1990); Tosun *et al.* (2008); Smidt and van der Windt (2006); Johnson *et al.* (2007); Brinker and Miller (1999); Leslie and Dickson (1981); Anderson (2011); McRae (2010); Atroshi *et al.* (1999); Silverstein, Fine and Armstrong (1987)

## Red Flags

Red flags help to identify serious pathology in patients with chronic pain. If a red flag symptom is found in a patient, the practitioner should exercise utmost caution and prioritise sound clinical reasoning, so that the patient is not placed at risk of an undue adverse event due to manipulation.

**Table 14.8 Red flags for serious pathology in the elbow, wrist and hand**

| Condition | Signs and symptoms |
|---|---|
| Compartment syndrome | <ul><li>History of trauma or surgery</li><li>Persistent forearm pain and tightness</li><li>Pain intensified with stretch applied to affected muscles</li><li>Increased tension in the involved compartment</li><li>Tingling, burning or numbness</li><li>Paraesthesia, paresis and sensory deficits</li><li>Symptoms unchanged by position or movement</li></ul> |
| Radial head fracture | <ul><li>History of fall on an outstretched arm</li><li>Radial head tenderness</li><li>High guard position of the upper extremity</li><li>Elbow joint effusion</li><li>Restricted or painful supination and pronation, active range of motion</li></ul> |
| Avascular necrosis | <ul><li>Pain and stiffness in the upper arm</li><li>Gradual onset of pain</li><li>History of excessive alcohol use</li><li>Prolonged use of oral steroids</li><li>Previous history of undergoing chemotherapy and radiation (less common)</li></ul> |
| Lunate fracture | <ul><li>Generalised wrist pain</li><li>History of a dorsiflexion injury of the hand or a fall on to an outstretched hand</li><li>Severe pain with gripping things or moving the wrist</li><li>Reduced grip strength</li></ul> |
| Scaphoid fracture | <ul><li>History of a fall on to an outstretched hand</li><li>Pain with or without swelling or bruising at the base of the thumb</li><li>Severe pain with grabbing or gripping things</li><li>Difficulty in moving and twisting the wrist or thumb</li><li>Reduced movement around the wrist</li></ul> |

| Condition | Signs and symptoms |
|---|---|
| Long flexor tendon rupture | • An injury on the palm side of the hand<br>• Numbness in the fingertip<br>• Pain with bending the finger<br>• Inability to move or bend one or more joints of the finger, such as DIP or PIP joint<br>• Forceful flexor contraction |
| Malignancy | • Asymmetric or irregular shape lesion<br>• Unexplained deformity, mass or swelling<br>• Chronic pain in bones<br>• Unexplained weight loss<br>• Extreme tiredness (fatigue)<br>• Repeated infection<br>• Persistent low-grade fever, either constant or intermittent |
| Infection | • Fever, chills, malaise and weakness<br>• Recent bacterial infection such as urinary tract or skin infection<br>• Recent cut, scrape or puncture wound<br>• Loss of appetite |

Sources: Harvey (2001); Jawed *et al.* (2001); Hunter, Mackin and Callahan (2002); Reiman (2016); Weinzweig and Gonzalez (2002); Phillips, Reibach and Slomiany (2004); Forman, Forman and Rose (2005)

## Special Tests

**Table 14.9 Special tests for assessing serious pathology in the elbow, wrist and hand**

| Test | Procedure | Positive sign | Interpretation |
|---|---|---|---|
| Varus stress test | The patient sits with elbow flexed to 15–20 degrees. The examiner stabilises the arm with one hand placed at the elbow and the other hand placed above the wrist. Finally, the examiner applies a varus force to the elbow. | Lateral (radial) pain and/or increased laxity when compared with uninvolved | ☐ Lateral collateral ligament injury |

| Valgus stress test | The patient sits with elbow flexed to 15–20 degrees. The examiner stabilises the arm with one hand placed at the elbow and the other hand placed above the wrist. Finally, the examiner applies a valgus force to the elbow. | Medial (ulnar) pain and/or increased laxity when compared with uninvolved | ☐ Medial collateral ligament injury |
|---|---|---|---|
| Tennis elbow test | The examiner stabilises the involved elbow with one hand and instructs the patient to make a fist, pronate the forearm, and radially deviate and extend the wrist against the examiner's resisting force at the fist. | Sharp, sudden or severe pain over the lateral humeral epicondyle | ☐ Lateral epicondylitis |
| Tinel's sign test | The patient is seated with the elbow in slight flexion. The examiner lightly taps the volar aspect of the patient's wrist over the median nerve. | Tingling or paraesthesia along the ulnar distribution of the forearm, hand and fingers | ☐ Ulnar nerve injury |
| Phalen's test | Examiner instructs the patient to hold wrists in a fully flexed position for 1–2 minutes. | Exacerbation of paraesthesia in the median nerve distribution | ☐ Carpal tunnel syndrome |
| Murphy's sign test | Examiner asks the patient to make a fist and then observes the position of the third metacarpal. | Third metacarpal head is level with the second and fourth metacarpal heads | ☐ Dislocated lunate |
| Flexor digitorum superficialis test | Examiner instructs the patient to flex the proximal interphalangeal joint of the involved finger while keeping the other fingers extended. | Inability to flex the proximal interphalangeal joint | ☐ Disrupted flexor digitorum superficialis |

| Test | Procedure | Positive sign | Interpretation |
|---|---|---|---|
| Flexor digitorum profundus test | Examiner instructs the patient to extend the distal interphalangeal joint of the involved finger while keeping the other fingers extended. | Inability to flex the distal interphalangeal joint | ☐ Disrupted flexor digitorum profundus |
| Allen's test | The examiner instructs the patient to make a tight fist and open it fully several times. The patient then squeezes fist to 'pump' the blood out of the hand and fingers. The examiner compresses the radial and ulnar arteries. The patient relaxes their hand and the examiner releases one artery at a time, observing the colour of the hand and fingers. | Failure of the radial or ulnar half of the hand to flush red immediately | ☐ Occlusion of radial or ulnar artery |

Sources: Baxter (2003); Cooper (2007); McRae (2010); Lynch (2004); Saunders *et al.* (2015)

# References

Alcid, J.G., Ahmad, C.S. and Lee, T.Q. (2004). Elbow anatomy and structural biomechanics. *Clinics in Sports Medicine, 23*(4), 503–517.

Anderson, D. (2011). Mallet finger: Management and patient compliance. *Australian Family Physician, 40*(1/2), 47.

Atroshi, I., Gummesson, C., Johnsson, R., Ornstein, E., Ranstam, J. and Rosén, I. (1999). Prevalence of carpal tunnel syndrome in a general population. *Journal of the American Medical Association, 282*(2), 153–158.

Baxter, R.E. (2003). *Pocket Guide to Musculoskeletal Assessment*. WB Saunders.

Brantingham, J.W., Cassa, T.K., Bonnefin, D., Pribicevic, M. *et al.* (2013). Manipulative and multimodal therapy for upper extremity and temporomandibular disorders: A systematic review. *Journal of Manipulative and Physiological Therapeutics, 36*(3), 143–201.

Brigstocke, G., Hearnden, A., Holt, C.A. and Whatling, G. (2013). The functional range of movement of the human wrist. *Journal of Hand Surgery (European Volume), 38*(5), 554–556.

Brinker, M.R. and Miller, M.D. (1999). *Fundamentals of Orthopaedics*. WB Saunders.

Bronfort, G., Haas, M., Evans, R., Leininger, B. and Triano, J. (2010). Effectiveness of manual therapies: The UK evidence report. *Chiropractic and Osteopathy, 18*(1), 1.

Cooper, G. (2007). *Pocket Guide to Musculoskeletal Diagnosis.* Springer Science & Business Media.

Doyle, J.R. (Ed.) (2003). *Surgical Anatomy of the Hand and Upper Extremity.* Philadelphia, PA: Lippincott Williams & Wilkins.

Ernst, E. (2007). Adverse effects of spinal manipulation: A systematic review. *Journal of the Royal Society of Medicine, 100*(7), 330–338.

Floyd, R.T. and Thompson, C.W. (2004). *Manual of Structural Kinesiology.* New York, NY: McGraw-Hill.

Forman, T.A., Forman, S.K. and Rose, N.E. (2005). A clinical approach to diagnosing wrist pain. *American Family Physician, 72*(9), 1753–1758.

Fornalski, S., Gupta, R. and Lee, T.Q. (2003). Anatomy and biomechanics of the elbow joint. *Techniques in Hand and Upper Extremity Surgery, 7*(4), 168–178.

Harvey, C. (2001). Compartment syndrome: When it is least expected. *Orthopaedic Nursing, 20*(3), 15–25.

Hunter, J.M., Mackin, E.J. and Callahan, A.D. (2002). *Rehabilitation of the Hand and Upper Extremity,* 5th edition. Mosby.

Jawed, S., Jawad, A.S.M., Padhiar, N. and Perry, J.D. (2001). Chronic exertional compartment syndrome of the forearms secondary to weight training. *Rheumatology, 40*(3), 344–345.

Johnson, G.W., Cadwallader, K., Scheffel, S.B. and Epperly, T.D. (2007). Treatment of lateral epicondylitis. *American Family Physician, 76*(6), 843–848.

Kuxhaus, L. (2008). *Development of a Feedback-Controlled Elbow Simulator: Design Validation and Clinical Application.* Ann Arbor, MI: ProQuest.

Lason, G. and Peeters, L. (2014). *The Elbow, Wrist and Hand.* The International Academy of Osteopathy.

Leslie, I.J. and Dickson, R.A. (1981). The fractured carpal scaphoid. Natural history and factors influencing outcome. *Journal of Bone and Joint Surgery, 63*(2), 225 230.

Lynch, J.M. (2004). Hand and wrist injuries: Part I. Nonemergent evaluation. *American Family Physician, 69*(8), 1941–1948.

McCann, S. and Wise, E. (2011). *Kaplan Anatomy Coloring Book.* Kaplan Publishing.

McHardy, A., Hoskins, W., Pollard, H., Onley, R. and Windsham, R. (2008). Chiropractic treatment of upper extremity conditions: A systematic review. *Journal of Manipulative and Physiological Therapeutics, 31*(2), 146–159.

McRae, R., 2010. *Clinical Orthopaedic Examination.* Elsevier Health Sciences.

Morrey, B.F., Askew, L.J. and Chao, E.Y. (1981). A biomechanical study of normal functional elbow motion. *The Journal of Bone and Joint Surgery, 63*(6), 872–877.

Nelson, D.L., Mitchell, M.A., Groszewski, P.G., Pennick, S.L. and Manske, P.R. (1994). Wrist range of motion in activities of daily living. In: *Advances in the Biomechanics of the Hand and Wrist.* Springer US.

Norkin, C.C. and White, D.J. (2009). *Measurement of Joint Motion: A Guide to Goniometry.* FA Davis.

Ootes, D., Lambers, K.T. and Ring, D.C. (2012). The epidemiology of upper extremity injuries presenting to the emergency department in the United States. *Hand, 7*(1), 18–22.

Ovesen, O., Brok, K.E., Arreskøv, J. and Bellstrøm, T. (1990). Monteggia lesions in children and adults: An analysis of etiology and long-term results of treatment. *Orthopedics, 13*(5), 529–534.

Paterson, J.K. and Burn, L. (2012). *An Introduction to Medical Manipulation*. Springer Science & Business Media.

Phillips, T.G., Reibach, A.M. and Slomiany, W.P. (2004). Diagnosis and management of scaphoid fractures. *American Family Physician, 70*, 879–892.

Reiman, M.P. (2016). *Orthopedic Clinical Examination*. Human Kinetics.

Saunders, R., Astifidis, R., Burke, S.L., Higgins, J. and McClinton, M.A. (2015). *Hand and Upper Extremity Rehabilitation: A Practical Guide*. Elsevier Health Sciences.

Silverstein, B.A., Fine, L.J. and Armstrong, T.J. (1987). Occupational factors and carpal tunnel syndrome. *American Journal of Industrial Medicine, 11*(3), 343–358.

Smidt, N. and van der Windt, D.A. (2006). Tennis elbow in primary care: Corticosteroid injections provide only short term pain relief. *British Medical Journal, 333*(7575), 927 –928.

Standring, S. (2008). *Gray's Anatomy: The Anatomical Basis of Clinical Practice*. London: Churchill Livingstone.

Tosun, B., Selek, O., Buluc, L. and Memisoglu, K. (2008). Chronic post-traumatic radial head dislocation associated with dissociation of distal radio-ulnar joint: A case report. *Archives of Orthopaedic and Trauma Surgery, 128*(7), 669–671.

Vasen, A.P., Lacey, S.H., Keith, M.W. and Shaffer, J.W. (1995). Functional range of motion of the elbow. *The Journal of Hand Surgery, 20*(2), 288–292.

Villaseñor-Ovies, P., Vargas, A., Chiapas-Gasca, K., Canoso, J.J. *et al.* (2012). Clinical anatomy of the elbow and shoulder. *Reumatología Clínica, 8*, 13–24

Weinzweig, N. and Gonzalez, M. (2002). Surgical infections of the hand and upper extremity: A county hospital experience. *Annals of Plastic Surgery, 49*(6), 621–627.

Whiteside, J.A., Andrews, J.R. and Fleisig, G.S. (1999). Elbow injuries in young baseball players. *The Physician and Sports Medicine, 27*(6), 87–102.

World Health Organization (2005). *WHO Guidelines on Basic Training and Safety in Chiropractic*. Geneva: World Health Organization.

# Techniques for the Elbow, Wrist and Hand

## Radial Head Manipulation

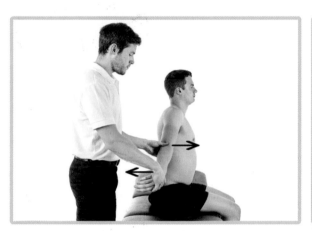 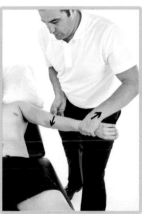

- The technique can be applied supine, seated or recumbent.
- Stand on the side of the arm to be manipulated as shown.
- You should stand with an asymmetrical stance.
- Locate and palpate the lateral aspect of the radial head.
- With your other hand, grasp around the patient's wrist and pronate the forearm to 45° (so their thumb is now facing downwards).
- Engage the barrier and perform the manipulation by pronating the forearm, flexing the wrist and fully extending the elbow while applying pressure to the radial head, moving it obliquely.

**Key Points**
- You can flex the elbow to 90°, with the arm closest palpating the radial head and the other hand on the wrist creating pronation and supination to help locate it.
- You can assess how much extension is available in the target elbow beforehand, and stand with your abdomen closer to the patient, enabling a barrier to prevent hyperextension during the manipulation.
- Avoid hyperextension of the patient's elbow.

## Ulna – Humeral Manipulation – Olecranon Contact

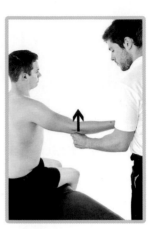

- The technique is performed supine, seated or recumbent.
- You stand to the side of the target joint.
- Support the medial and lateral epicondyle of the humerus with your thumb and second finger by forming a semi-clenched fist.
- Your other hand grasps around the patient's wrist, as shown.
- The manipulation is generated by your right hand extending the elbow via the wrist and simultaneously moving the dominant hand superiorly as shown, pressing into the medial and lateral humeral condyles.

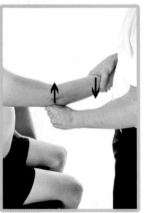

**Key Point**

- Avoid hyperextension of the elbow.

## Carpal Manipulation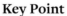

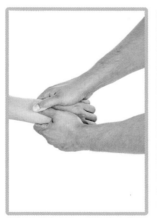
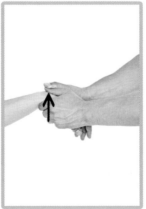
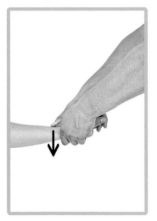

- The technique can be applied supine, seated or recumbent.
- Stand at side of table facing towards the patient.

- Hold the patient's fully pronated hand with both hands as shown.
- Locate the desired carpal bone to manipulate and cross your thumbs over it.
- Flex and extend patient's wrist with momentum.
- The manipulation is directed towards the palmar aspect of the hand as you move the wrist into extension.

### Key Points

- Spreading the hypothenar and thenar muscles enables greater potential for carpal dorsal movement.
- Numerous levers can be applied prior to extension (i.e. traction, radial/ulnar deviation flexion/extension to wrist).
- This technique is appropriate for all carpal bones.

## 1st Metacarpal Manipulation

- The technique can be applied supine, seated or recumbent.
- With your right hand, hold the patient's thumb as shown.
- Your thumb then palpates the groove between the base of the proximal 1st metacarpal joint and the trapezium.
- Your thumb fixes down in the plateau between the 1st metacarpal joint and the trapezium.
- Use your hand to grip and traction the 1st metacarpal – this will open the joint space of the 1st metacarpal – then place your application (manipulating thumb, as shown) over the joint line.
- Place your palmar surface over your other hand, reinforcing the posterior surface of your 1st metacarpal phalangeal joint.

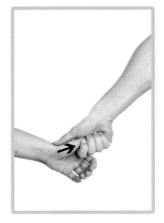

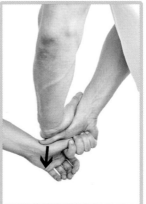

- You can extend your arms slightly, creating extension and traction applied to the patient's proximal end of their 1st metacarpal joint.
- The patient is then asked to inhale and exhale.
- As the patient exhales, engage the barrier.
- As the patient exhales, manipulate downwards as shown.

**Key Points**
- You can ask the patient to lean backwards to enhance the traction.
- Do not use excessive force.

## 1st Metacarpal Manipulation Variation

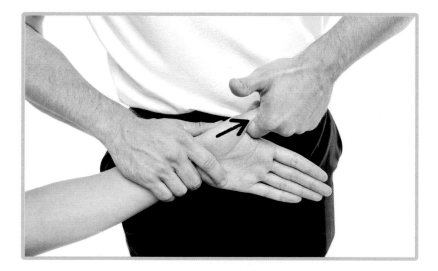

- The technique can be applied supine, seated or recumbent.
- Stand on the same side that you intend to manipulate.
- Your right hand holds the patient's wrist, securing the carpals.
- With the same hand, palpate the groove between the base of the proximal 1st metacarpal joint and the trapezium.
- Your left hand holds the 1st metacarpal phalangeal joint.
- You then add traction to the 1st metacarpal phalangeal joint.
- Internally rotate the 1st metacarpal.
- With traction and internal rotation being applied to the 1st metacarpal, the manipulation is achieved with bilateral extension of your arms.

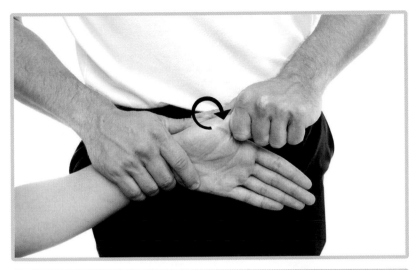

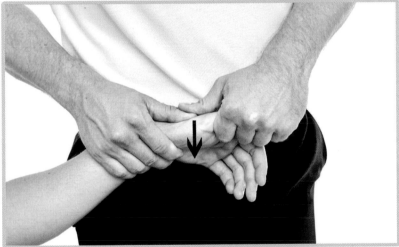

**Key Point**
- Even when manipulating the peripheral joints, work with the patient's breathing.

CHAPTER 15

# The Knee, Ankle and Foot

## Introduction

From the 19th century onwards, the use of manual therapy to treat various musculoskeletal conditions has increased progressively. Although it is still considered a relatively new approach to balance the bones and soft-tissue structures of the body, the use of manipulative techniques, in fact, predates Hippocrates (Dananberg, Shearstone and Guillano, 2000). Today, manual therapy has most commonly been used for the treatment of spinal pathologies, particularly low back pain. However, it has also been successful in treating many structures of the musculoskeletal system, including restrictions at the foot as well as proximal joints (knee and ankle) (Dananberg, 2004).

A number of promising studies have recently indicated that both joint manipulation and soft-tissue mobilisation may significantly improve restricted knee and ankle range of motion (ROM), and provide superior short-term relief from heel and toe pain (Mohammed, Syed and Ahmed, 2009; Andersen, Fryer and McLaughlin, 2003; Grieve *et al.*, 2011; Cleland *et al.*, 2009; Renan-Ordine *et al.*, 2011). Advocates of manual therapy believe that a great majority of patients with knee, ankle and foot pathologies can benefit from joint mobilisations and soft-tissue techniques. In addition, they claim that these techniques are comparatively safe and effective when compared with conventional interventions (Paterson and Burn, 2012).

Practitioners of manual therapy utilise a wide range of mobilising and manipulation techniques depending on the knee, ankle and foot joints and/or lesions being treated. The therapeutic goal of these practitioners is to apply a procedure that is well tolerated by the recipient and yields the best result. They primarily aim to adjust malalignment of bony and soft-tissue structures, improve mobility and function, and strengthen the surrounding muscles (Whitmore, Gladney and Driver, 2005; Brantingham *et al.*, 2012).

However, before deciding to apply manipulative techniques to the knee, ankle and foot joints, a practitioner must make sure that no red flags or contraindications are present (Rivett, Thomas and Bolton, 2005). In addition, because adequate knowledge and skill, good handling and proper use of body posture are imperative to apply these techniques accurately and effectively, practitioners must rehearse the techniques repeatedly to apply them with confidence and control in clinical practice (Domholdt, 2000; Hodges and Gandevia, 2000; Dunne, 2001). It is also essential for practitioners to have a thorough understanding of anatomy and body biomechanics, so that they can accurately palpate bony surface landmarks. Therefore, practitioners should have appropriate training and education before they start applying these techniques to their patients (Di Fabio, 1992; World Health Organization, 2005).

The purpose of this chapter is to help practitioners diagnose serious pathologies in the knee, ankle and foot regions. This chapter describes the various joints of these structures, the range of motion in their joints, some common injuries to the regions and the red flags for manipulation.

## Joints

In human anatomy, the knee is one of the largest joints in the human body. It comprises bones, cartilage, ligaments and tendons. The knee joint connects the upper and lower leg bones, and is the anatomical region where four bones – the femur, tibia, fibula and patella – meet. Apart from the fibula, these bones are all functional in the knee joint (Tate, 2009).

On the other hand, the ankle and foot are the most distal parts of the lower limb. The bones, ligaments, tendons and muscles of the ankle and foot are highly developed, complex structures. The joints of the ankle and foot are functionally different compared with other joints in the body, because they are at times mobile and at other times quite stable. These structures serve the body by providing mobility and stability, and play diverse roles in our activities of daily living (Riegger, 1988).

**Table 15.1 The joints of the knee, ankle and foot**

| Joint name | Description | Function |
|---|---|---|
| Knee joint | <ul><li>A synovial (modified hinge) joint, consisting of three distinct and partially separated compartments</li><li>Forms a complex hinge between three bones: the femur, the tibia and the patella</li><li>Involves two separate articulations: one joining the tibia and femur (tibiofemoral joint), and another joining the patella and femur (patellofemoral joint)</li><li>Surrounded by a single articular capsule that encloses the entire joint complex</li></ul> | <ul><li>Ensures weight-bearing support by allowing flexion and extension of the leg</li><li>Allows transmission of body weight in vertical and horizontal directions</li><li>Permits a small amount of internal and external rotation when flexed</li></ul> |
| Tibiofemoral joint | <ul><li>A synovial hinge-type joint</li><li>Connects the medial and lateral condyles of the femur (thigh bone) with the medial and lateral condyles of the tibia</li><li>Supported by two wedge-shaped articular discs: the medial meniscus and lateral meniscus</li></ul> | <ul><li>Serves as the weight-bearing joint of the knee</li><li>Allows flexion and extension of the knee</li></ul> |
| Patellofemoral joint | <ul><li>A saddle-type complex joint of the knee that is often misunderstood</li><li>Formed by joining the anterior and distal part of the femur with the patella (kneecap)</li></ul> | <ul><li>Allows the knee to straighten when standing</li><li>Helps to perform the activities of daily living</li></ul> |

| Superior tibiofibular joint | • A plane-type synovial joint formed by joining the lateral edge of the tibia with the head of the fibula<br>• Composed of two facet joints: one on the posterolateral aspect of the tibial condyle and one on the medial upper surfaces of the head of the fibula | • Dissipates torsional stresses applied at the ankle<br>• Dissipates lateral tibial bending movements |
|---|---|---|
| Inferior tibiofibular joint | • A syndesmosis formed by joining the distal end of the fibula with the lateral side of the tibia<br>• Is supported by strong interosseus ligament | • Permits slight movements to allow the lateral malleolus to rotate laterally when the ankle dorsiflexes<br>• Helps to maintain the ankle joint integrity |
| Ankle or talocrural joint | • A hinge joint formed superiorly by the distal tibia and fibula and inferiorly by the dome of the talus<br>• Involves articulation between three bones (the tibia, fibula and talus)<br>• Is supported by strong ligamentous structures that provides stability to the ankle | • Allows dorsiflexion and plantar flexion movements via axis in talus |
| Subtalar or talocalcaneal joint | • A modified multiaxial joint formed between two of the tarsal bones: the talus and the calcaneus (heel bone)<br>• Involves three articulations between talus and calcaneus: anterior, middle and posterior | • Permits inversion and eversion motions of the foot |
| Talocalcaneo-navicular joint | • A compound, multiaxial joint formed when the rounded head of the talus connects with the navicular and the calcaneus<br>• Includes two articulations: an anterior talocalcaneal and a talonavicular | • Allows plantar flexion of talus on the navicular |
| Calcaneocuboid joint | • A biaxial joint that is considered among the least mobile joints of the foot<br>• Involves articulation between the heel bone and the cuboid bone | • Allows a movement, which is best referred to as obvolution-involution |

| Joint name | Description | Function |
|---|---|---|
| Tarsometatarsal or lisfranc joints | • Arthrodial joints that are formed between the tarsal bones of the mid-foot (the 1st, 2nd and 3rd cuneiform bones and the cuboid bone) and the bases of the metatarsal bones<br>• Are strengthened by strong interosseus dorsal, and plantar ligaments | • Allow slight gliding movements at the feet |
| Intermetatarsal joints | • Synovial joints that involve articulations between the bases of the metatarsal bones<br>• Are strengthened by strong interosseus dorsal and plantar ligaments | • Allow slight gliding movements at the feet |
| Metatarsopha-langeal joints | • Ellipsoid joints formed by joining the heads of the metatarsal bones with the bases of the proximal bones (proximal phalanges)<br>• Are strengthened by collateral and plantar ligaments | • Allow a variety of movements at the toes, including flexion, extension, abduction, adduction and circumduction |
| Interphalangeal joints | • Ginglymoid (hinge) joints formed by the articulations between the superior surfaces on the phalangeal heads and the adjacent phalangeal bases<br>• Subdivided into two sets of articulations: proximal interphalangeal joints and distal interphalangeal joints | • Permit flexion and extension movements |

Sources: Tate (2009); McCann and Wise (2011); Standring (2008); Riegger (1988); Norkin and White (2009)

## Range of Motion

### Knee

The knee joint is well constructed for the transmission of body weight in vertical and horizontal directions. It allows flexion and extension, with slight internal and external rotation about the axis of the lower leg in the flexed position. The stability and normal movements at the knee are essential for performing many daily activities, including walking, running, kicking, sitting and standing (Mader, 2004). The range of motion of the knee is typically measured using a hand goniometer. However, visual estimation and radiographic goniometry are also used to measure the range of motion.

**Table 15.2 Normal range of motion of the knee**

| Movement type | Range of motion |
|---|---|
| Flexion | 120–150° |
| Extension | 5–10° |
| Lateral rotation (knee flexed 90°) | 30–40° |
| Medial rotation (knee flexed 90°) | 10° |

Source: Schünke *et al.* (2006)

**Table 15.3 Range of motion of the knee in different age groups (in degrees)**

| Age | Motion | Males | Females |
|---|---|---|---|
| 2–8 years | Flexion | 147.8 (146.6–149.0) | 152.6 (151.2–154.0) |
| | Extension | 1.6 (0.9–2.3) | 5.4 (3.9–6.9) |
| 9–19 years | Flexion | 142.2 (140.4–44.0) | 142.3 (140.8–143.8) |
| | Extension | 1.8 (0.9–2.7) | 2.4 (1.5–3.3) |
| 20–44 years | Flexion | 137.7 (136.5–138.9) | 141.9 (140.9–142.9) |
| | Extension | 1.0 (0.6–1.4) | 1.6 (1.1–2.1) |
| 45–69 years | Flexion | 132.9 (131.6–134.2) | 137.8 (136.5–139.1) |
| | Extension | 0.5 (0.1–0.9) | 1.2 (0.7–1.7) |

Numeric variables expressed as degree (range).

Source: Soucie *et al.* (2011)

### Ankle

The ankle allows dorsiflexion and plantar flexion movements at the foot. However, the axis of rotation of the ankle is dynamic because of the complex morphology of the talocrural joint.

**Table 15.4 Approximate range of motion of the ankle**

| Movement type | Range of motion | Reference |
|---|---|---|
| Normal dorsiflexion | 0–50° | Clarkson (2000) |
| Normal plantar flexion | 0–20° | |
| Dorsiflexion, knee extended | 14–48° | Spink *et al.* (2011) |
| Dorsiflexion, knee flexed | 16–60° | |

### Foot

The movement of the foot joints is complex. The motion of the subtalar joint is triplanar. It permits pronation and supination movements and allows 1° of freedom. The transverse tarsal joint, though, permits some degrees of inversion and eversion motions, but it mainly serves to amplify the motions of the talocrural joint and the subtalar joint (Oatis, 1988). The motion of the tarsometatarsal joints is translatory or planar. They continue the compensatory movement produced at the transverse tarsal joint when it reaches its maximum range of motion. The metatarsophalangeal joints allow 2° of freedom, providing motion in the sagittal and transverse planes. The interphalangeal (IP) joints permit motion in the sagittal plane, allowing pure flexion and extension (Norkin and White, 2009).

**Table 15.5 Range of motion of the foot joints**

| Joint name | Movement type | Range of motion |
|---|---|---|
| Subtalar joint | Inversion | 0–50° |
| | Eversion | 0–26° |

| Metatarsophalangeal joints | Flexion (great toe) | 0–45° |
| | Extension (great toe) | 0–80° |
| | Flexion (lesser toes) | 0–40° |
| | Extension (lesser toes) | 0–70° |
| Interphalangeal joints | Flexion (great toe) | 0–90° |
| | Flexion (lesser toes) | 0–30° |
| | Extension (great toe and other toes) | 0–80° |

Sources: Oatis (1988); Norkin and White (2009)

## Common Injuries

Knee, ankle and foot injuries are the most common musculoskeletal injuries. Most injuries to these regions are caused by a fall, motor vehicle accident, violent activity, sport accident or penetrating trauma. These injuries are common in all populations, including male and female, the very young and the old, and participants of numerous sports. In athletes, the knee, ankle and foot are the most commonly injured parts of the body. These injuries are linked to both short-term and long-term disability and can significantly upset activities of daily living.

**Table 15.6 Common injuries of the knee, ankle and foot**

| Injury | Characteristics |
|---|---|
| Anterior cruciate ligament sprain | • One of the most common knee injuries<br>• Involves tearing of the anterior cruciate ligament – a ligament that keeps the knee stable<br>• Occurs most commonly in athletes who actively participate in demanding sports such as football, soccer, tennis, downhill skiing, volleyball and basketball<br>• Often occurs with a 'popping' noise<br>• Causes include slowing down when running, rapid changing of direction, stopping suddenly or landing from a jump<br>• About 50% of these injuries potentially damage other structures in the knee, including meniscus, articular cartilage or other ligaments |

| Injury | Characteristics |
|---|---|
| Medial collateral ligament sprain | • One of the most commonly injured ligaments of the knee<br>• Involves tearing of the medial collateral ligament – a ligament that prevents the knee from bending inward<br>• Occurs most commonly in athletes who participate in contact sports such as wrestling, judo, rugby, hockey and football<br>• Often occurs due to a hit or direct blow to the outer aspect of the knee<br>• Common causes include bending, twisting or rapid changing of direction while running<br>• Symptoms include a 'popping' noise, pain, swelling, tenderness and locking or catching in the knee |
| Meniscal tear | • One of the most common injuries to the knee<br>• Involves rupturing of the meniscus – a rubbery, C-shaped fibrocartilaginous structure that cushions the knee<br>• Common causes include forceful twisting, quick turning or hyperflexion of the knee joint<br>• High-risk group: individuals who participate in contact sports<br>• Symptoms include pain, swelling, a 'popping' noise and tenderness in the knee<br>• Accounts for nearly 11% of all knee injuries |
| Patellar tendonitis | • An inflammation of the patellar tendon at the inferior patellar region or at the insertion of the quadriceps tendon at the base of the patella<br>• Occurs most commonly in teenage boys, particularly in athletes who actively participate in jumping sports<br>• Often associated with excessive foot pronation, patellar malalignment or patella alta<br>• Symptoms include anterior knee pain and localised swelling, thickening or nodules |
| Ankle sprain | • The most common injury to the ankle<br>• Involves stretching of the strong ankle ligaments beyond their limits and, possibly, tearing them<br>• High-risk group: individuals who participate in forceful athletic activities, which require rapid shifting of movement, such as such as running and jumping sports<br>• Linked to both short-term and long-term disability<br>• Rate of incidence: 61 per 10,000 individuals in the UK |

| | |
|---|---|
| Plantar fasciitis | • A degenerative disease of the plantar fascia<br>• The most common cause of stabbing pain in the heel and bottom of the foot<br>• Commonly affects middle-aged people<br>• About 10% of individuals develop it at some stage during their lifetime<br>• Risk factors include leg length inconsistency, nerve entrapment, muscle tightness, excessive pronation, over-training and using ill-fitting footwear |
| Peroneal tendonitis | • The most common overuse injury that causes ankle pain at the lateral portion<br>• Causes inflammation of the peroneal tendons<br>• Often occurs as a result of excessive eversion and pronation<br>• Commonly affects athletes, particularly those who are involved in repetitive ankle motion |

Sources: Frontera (2015); Roach *et al.* (2014); Rodkey (1999); Nicholl, Coleman and Williams (1991); Calmbach and Hutchens (2003a); O'Loughlin *et al.* (2009); Beeson (2014); Wang *et al.* (2005)

# Red Flags

Red flags help to identify serious pathology in patients with chronic pain. If a red flag symptom is found in a patient, the practitioner should exercise utmost caution and prioritise sound clinical reasoning, so that the patient is not placed at risk of an undue adverse event due to manipulation.

**Table 15.7 Red flags for serious pathology in the knee, ankle, and foot**

| Condition | Signs and symptoms |
|---|---|
| Knee fractures | • History of recent trauma such as a knee injury or a fall from height<br>• Pain, bruising or swelling on affected leg<br>• Numbness, tingling or a pins-and-needles sensation<br>• Difficulty in bending the knee<br>• Inability to walk or bear weight on involved leg |

| Compartment syndrome | • History of trauma<br>• Severe, persistent pain and hardness to anterior compartment of shin<br>• Pain with dorsiflexion of toes<br>• Pain intensifies with stretch applied to affected muscles<br>• Swelling, tightness and bruising of involved compartment |
|---|---|
| Extensor mechanism disruption | • Ruptured quadriceps or patella tendon<br>• Altered position of the patella (superior translation) |
| Fractures | • History of recent trauma such as a crush injury, an ankle injury or a fall from height<br>• Pain, bruising or swelling on affected leg<br>• Persistent synovitis<br>• Point tenderness over involved tissues<br>• Inability to walk or bear weight on involved leg |
| Deep vein thrombosis | • History of recent surgery<br>• Calf pain<br>• Redness of the skin<br>• Swelling and tenderness on affected leg<br>• Pain intensified with walking or standing and reduced by elevation and rest |
| Septic arthritis | • Fever, chills<br>• Recent bacterial infection, surgery or injection<br>• Severe, constant pain<br>• Systemically unwell such as unusual fatigue (malaise) or loss of appetite<br>• Coexisting immunosuppressive disorder<br>• Red, swollen joint with no history of trauma |
| Cancer | • Unremitting pain<br>• Previous history of cancer<br>• Atypical symptoms with no history of a trauma<br>• Systematic symptoms such as fever, chills, malaise and weakness<br>• Unexplained weight loss<br>• Suspected malignancy or unexplained deformity, mass or swelling |

Sources: McGee and Boyko (1998); Judd and Kim (2002); Gupta, Sturrock and Field (2001); Ulmer (2002)

## Special Tests

### Table 15.8 Special tests for assessing serious pathology in the knee, ankle and foot

| Test | Procedure | Positive sign | Interpretation |
|------|-----------|---------------|----------------|
| Lachman's test | The patient lies supine and the injured knee is flexed 20–30 degrees. The examiner stabilises the distal femur with one hand and holds the proximal tibia with the other hand. The examiner then applies a gentle anterior force to pull up on the tibia anteriorly. | • Excessive displacement of the tibia compared with the uninvolved knee | ☐ Compromised anterior cruciate ligament |
| Posterior drawer test | The patient lies supine with the hip flexed 45 degrees, the knee flexed 90 degrees and the tibia in neutral rotation. The examiner stabilises the patient's foot and pushes posteriorly on the tibia. | • Posterior displacement of the tibia with respect to the femur | ☐ Compromised posterior cruciate ligament |
| Valgus stress test | The patient lies supine. The examiner holds the lateral aspect of the patient's knee joint with one hand and places the other hand on the medial aspect of the distal tibia. Next, the examiner gently applies valgus stress on the knee at both zero degrees (full extension) and 30 degrees of flexion. | • Laxity of the medial collateral ligament on valgus stress | ☐ Compromised posterior and medial cruciate ligaments |

| Test | Procedure | Positive sign | Interpretation |
|---|---|---|---|
| McMurray's test | The patient lies supine. The examiner grasps the patient's heel with one hand and places the other hand on the knee, palpating the joint line (medial and lateral). To test the lateral meniscus, the examiner rotates the tibia internally and extends the knee from full flexion to 90 degrees. A varus stress is applied across the knee joint while the examiner extends the knee. To test the medial meniscus, the examiner rotates the tibia externally and extends the knee from full flexion to 90 degrees. A valgus stress is applied across the knee joint while the knee is being extended. | • Palpable click or pop and pain along joint line | ☐ Meniscal tears |
| Talar tilt test | The patient is seated with the ankle unsupported and the foot in 10–20 degrees of plantarflexed position. The examiner stabilises the distal lower leg, just proximal to medial malleolus, with one hand and applies an inversion force to the hindfoot with the other hand. The examiner tilts the talus side to side during inversion of the foot. | • Increased joint laxity or increased talar tilt compared with the contralateral side | ☐ Compromised calcaneofibular ligament |
| Thompson test | The patient lies prone, with the knee bent to 90 degrees. The examiner squeezes the calf muscle and looks for presence of ankle plantar flexion. | • Absence of ankle plantar flexion | ☐ Ruptured Achilles tendon |

| Anterior drawer test | The patient lies prone on the table, with the ankle in a neutral position and foot in 20 degrees of plantarflexed position. The examiner stabilises the distal tibia with one hand and applies an anterior force to the calcaneus (heel) with the other hand. | • Increased anterior translation compared to the contralateral side | ☐ Compromised anterior talofibular ligament |
|---|---|---|---|
| Kleiger's test | The patient is seated, with the knee flexed over the edge of the table by 90 degrees. The examiner stabilises the distal tibia with one hand and applies a rotational force externally to the affected foot. | • Medial and lateral joint pain or tibiofibular joint pain | ☐ Damage to distal tibiofibular syndesmosis<br>☐ Compromised deltoid ligament |

Sources: Baxter (2003); Calmbach and Hutchens (2003b); Hartley (1995); Young *et al.* (2005); Simpson and Howard (2009)

# References

Andersen, S., Fryer, G.A. and McLaughlin, P. (2003). The effect of talo-crural joint manipulation on range of motion at the ankle joint in subjects with a history of ankle injury. *Australasian Chiropractic and Osteopathy,* 11(2), 57.

Baxter, R.E. (2003). *Pocket Guide to Musculoskeletal Assessment.* WB Saunders.

Beeson, P. (2014). Plantar fasciopathy: Revisiting the risk factors. *Foot and Ankle Surgery,* 20(3), 160–165.

Brantingham, J.W., Bonnefin, D., Perle, S.M., Cassa, T.K. *et al.* (2012). Manipulative therapy for lower extremity conditions: Update of a literature review. *Journal of Manipulative and Physiological Therapeutics,* 35(2), 127–166.

Calmbach, W.L. and Hutchens, M. (2003a). Evaluation of patients presenting with knee pain: Part I. History, physical examination, radiographs, and laboratory tests. *American Family Physician,* 68(5), 907–912.

Calmbach, W.L. and Hutchens, M. (2003b). Evaluation of patients presenting with knee pain: Part II. Differential diagnosis. *American Family Physician,* 68(5), 917–922.

Clarkson, H.M. (2000). *Musculoskeletal Assessment: Joint Range of Motion and Manual Muscle Strength.* Philadelphia, PA: Lippincott Williams & Wilkins.

Cleland, J.A., Abbott, J.H., Kidd, M.O., Stockwell, S. *et al.* (2009). Manual physical therapy and exercise versus electrophysical agents and exercise in the management of plantar heel pain: A multicenter randomized clinical trial. *Journal of Orthopaedic and Sports Physical Therapy, 39*(8), 573–585.

Dananberg, H.J. (2004). Manipulation of the ankle as a method of treatment for ankle and foot pain. *Journal of the American Podiatric Medical Association, 94*(4), 395–399.

Dananberg, H.J., Shearstone, J. and Guillano, M. (2000). Manipulation method for the treatment of ankle equinus. *Journal of the American Podiatric Medical Association, 90*(8), 385–389.

Di Fabio, R.P. (1992). Efficacy of manual therapy. *Physical Therapy, 72*(12), 853–864.

Domholdt, E. (2000). *Physical Therapy Research: Principles and Applications.* WB Saunders Company.

Dunne, J. (2001). Pre-manipulative testing: Predicting risk or pretending to? *Australian Journal of Physiotherapy, 47*(3), 165.

Frontera, W.R. (2015). *Anterior Cruciate Ligament Tear. Essentials of Physical Medicine and Rehabilitation: Musculoskeletal Disorders, Pain, and Rehabilitation.* Philadelphia, PA: Saunders Elsevier.

Grieve, R., Clark, J., Pearson, E., Bullock, S., Boyer, C. and Jarrett, A. (2011). The immediate effect of soleus trigger point pressure release on restricted ankle joint dorsiflexion: A pilot randomised controlled trial. *Journal of Bodywork and Movement Therapies, 15*(1), 42–49.

Gupta, M.N., Sturrock, R.D. and Field, M. (2001). A prospective 2-year study of 75 patients with adult-onset septic arthritis. *Rheumatology, 40*(1), 24–30.

Hartley, A. (1995). *Practical Joint Assessment: Lower Quadrant: A Sports Medicine Manual,* Mosby-Year Book.

Hodges, P.W. and Gandevia, S.C. (2000). Activation of the human diaphragm during a repetitive postural task. *The Journal of Physiology, 522*(1), 165–175.

Judd, D.B. and Kim, D.H. (2002). Foot fractures frequently misdiagnosed as ankle sprains. *American Family Physician, 66*(5), 785–794.

Mader, S.S, (2004). *Understanding Human Anatomy and Physiology.* McGraw-Hill Science.

McCann, S. and Wise, E. (2011). *Kaplan Anatomy Coloring Book.* Kaplan Publishing.

McGee, S.R. and Boyko, E.J. (1998). Physical examination and chronic lower-extremity ischemia: A critical review. *Archives of Internal Medicine, 158*(12), 1357–1364.

Mohammed, R., Syed, S. and Ahmed, N. (2009). Manipulation under anaesthesia for stiffness following knee arthroplasty. *Annals of the Royal College of Surgeons of England, 91*(3), 220.

Nicholl, J.P., Coleman, P. and Williams, B.T. (1991). Pilot study of the epidemiology of sports injuries and exercise-related morbidity. *British Journal of Sports Medicine, 25*(1), 61–66.

Norkin, C.C. and White, D.J. (2009). *Measurement of Joint Motion: A Guide to Goniometry.* FA Davis.

Oatis, C.A. (1988). Biomechanics of the foot and ankle under static conditions. *Physical Therapy, 68*(12), 1815–1821.

O'Loughlin, P.F., Murawski, C.D., Egan, C. and Kennedy, J.G. (2009). Ankle instability in sports. *The Physician and Sports Medicine, 37*(2), 93–103.

Paterson, J.K. and Burn, L. (2012). *An Introduction to Medical Manipulation*. Springer Science & Business Media.

Renan-Ordine, R., Alburquerque-Sendín, F., Rodrigues De Souza, D.P., Cleland, J.A. and Fernández-de-las-Peñas, C. (2011). Effectiveness of myofascial trigger point manual therapy combined with a self-stretching protocol for the management of plantar heel pain: A randomized controlled trial. *Journal of Orthopaedic and Sports Physical Therapy, 41*(2), 43–50.

Riegger, C.L. (1988). Anatomy of the ankle and foot. *Physical Therapy, 68*(12), 1802–1814.

Rivett, D.A., Thomas, L. and Bolton, B. (2005). Premanipulative testing: Where do we go from here? *New Zealand Journal of Physiotherapy, 33*(3), 78–84.

Roach, C.J., Haley, C.A., Cameron, K.L., Pallis, M., Svoboda, S.J. and Owens, B.D. (2014). The epidemiology of medial collateral ligament sprains in young athletes. *The American Journal of Sports Medicine, 42*(5), 1103–1109.

Rodkey, W.G. (1999). Basic biology of the meniscus and response to injury. *Instructional Course Lectures, 49*, 189–193.

Schünke, M., Ross, L. M., Schulte, E., Schumacher, U. and Lamperti, E.D. (2006). *Thieme Atlas of Anatomy: General Anatomy and Musculoskeletal System*. Thieme.

Simpson, M. R. and Howard, T.M. (2009). Tendinopathies of the foot and ankle. *American Family Physician, 80*(10), 107–1114.

Soucie, J.M., Wang, C., Forsyth, A., Funk, S. *et al.* (2011). Range of motion measurements: Reference values and a database for comparison studies. *Haemophilia, 17*(3), 500–507.

Spink, M.J., Fotoohabadi, M.R., Wee, E., Hill, K.D., Lord, S.R. and Menz, H.B. (2011). Foot and ankle strength, range of motion, posture, and deformity are associated with balance and functional ability in older adults. *Archives of Physical Medicine and Rehabilitation, 92*(1), 68–75.

Standring, S. (2008). *Gray's Anatomy: The Anatomical Basis of Clinical Practice*. Churchill Livingstone.

Tate, P. (2009). *Anatomy of Bones and Joints. Seeley's Principles of Anatomy and Physiology*. McGraw-Hill.

Ulmer, T. (2002). The clinical diagnosis of compartment syndrome of the lower leg: Are clinical findings predictive of the disorder? *Journal of Orthopaedic Trauma, 16*(8), 572–577.

Wang, X.T., Rosenberg, Z.S., Mechlin, M.B. and Schweitzer, M.E. (2005). Normal variants and diseases of the peroneal tendons and superior peroneal retinaculum: MR imaging features 1. *Radiographics, 25*(3), 587–602.

Whitmore, S., Gladney, K. and Driver, A. (2005). *The Lower Quadrant: A Workbook of Manual Therapy Technique*. Whitmore Physiotherapy Consulting.

World Health Organization (2005). *WHO Guidelines on Basic Training and Safety in Chiropractic*. Geneva: World Health Organization.

Young, C.C., Niedfeldt, M.W., Morris, G.A. and Eerkes, K.J. (2005). Clinical examination of the foot and ankle. *Primary Care: Clinics in Office Practice, 32*(1), 105–132.

# Techniques for the Knee, Ankle and Foot

## Fibular Head Manipulation

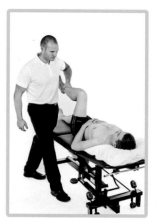
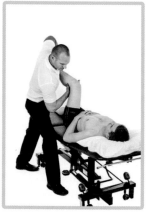
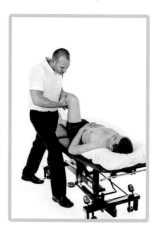
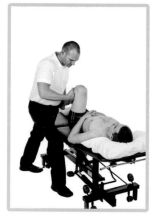
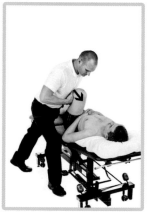

- The patient is in supine position.
- Stands on the side of the affected limb, facing the patient.
- Bend the patient's knee and hip to 90°.
- With the your left hand, hold the patient's distal tibia and fibula, and use this hand to control the movement needed.

- Place your right hand around the lateral aspect of the knee so that the 1st MCP joint is in contact with the posterior aspect of the proximal fibula head and the fingers are resting gently in the popliteal fossa.
- With your left hand, move the lower leg towards the patient's gluteal in an SI direction until you reach full knee flexion and the back of the contact hand is in contact with the tissues of the distal hamstrings.
- Ask the patient to inhale and exhale.
- At the end of the exhalation, engage the barrier and manipulate the fibula head AP.

**Key Points**
- Also in this position, you can stabilise the patient's lower leg by applying gentle pressure with your abdomen to the shin.
- The technique is used to increase PA movement in the fibula.
- Be aware that in patients with knees with limited flexion this technique may not be possible.
- Speed is key; the quicker the manipulation, the less force is needed.

# Fibula Head Manipulation Variation

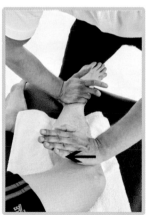

- This technique is performed with the patient lying on their side, with the affected fibular head uppermost.
- Bend the knees to 45 degrees and leave the superior leg to lie in front of the inferior leg on the table.
- Use an asymmetrical stance.
- Contact over the lateral malleolus with the pisiform of one hand. Place a downward pressure through the malleolus to secure the leg to the table.
- Your other hand should contact on to the superior surface of the fibula head.
- Ask the patient to inhale and exhale.
- At the end of the exhalation, engage the barrier and perform the manipulation variation.

### Key Points

- This technique is useful for patients who are unable to fully flex the knee.
- To ensure a firm contact, take a wider contact at first, and create skin-slack-drag across towards the contact.
- Swap the hands to allow for posterior and anterior movement of the fibula head.

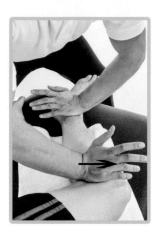

## Side-Lying Tibiotalar Manipulation

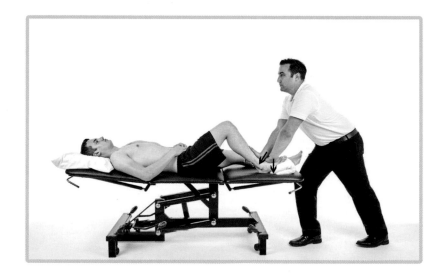

- Have the patient in a side-lying position with hip and knee flexed between 45°and 90°.
- For comfort, place a towel under the patient's tibia and foot.
- Position yourself at the foot of the table with an asymmetrical stance.
- Your right hand contacts the medial aspect of the calcaneus.
- Your left hand contacts the mid-foot. Your 1st MCP contacts the navicular and supinates the foot.
- Ask the patient to inhale and exhale.
- At the end of the exhalation, engage the barrier by increasing tension through both hands.

- Once the barrier is engaged, perform the manipulation with your right hand moving AP and IS; your left hand manipulates directly AP.

**Key Points**
- Creating supination of the foot directs manipulation to the desired joint while limiting the force of the manipulation to other joints of the foot.
- Use of a drop piece (if one is available with your bench) is very effective in this situation as it reduces the amount of force needed.

# Supine Tibiotalar Manipulation

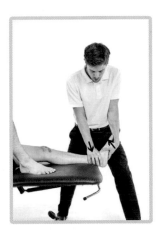

- The patient is in supine position with the foot just off the table as shown.
- For the patient's comfort, place a towel underneath the lower leg.
- Stand at the foot of the table with an asymmetrical stance, facing the foot as shown.
- Place your right hand, with a broad contact between the thumb and index finger, just inferior to the malleoli.
- Your left hand contacts around the plantar aspect of the foot with the fingers facing towards the floor.
- Ask the patient to inhale and exhale.
- At the end of exhalation, engage the barrier.
- Once the barrier is engaged, manipulate the joint by creating ML with your left hand.
- The stabilising hand does just that. There is no need to thrust with this hand.

**Key Points**
- Adjust the height of the table to allow you to contact the patient's foot with arms almost straight.
- The foot should be positioned so that the plantar aspect of the foot is resting against your forearm.

- Use of a drop piece (if one is available with your table) is very effective in this situation as it reduces the amount of force needed.

## Prone Tibiotalar Manipulation

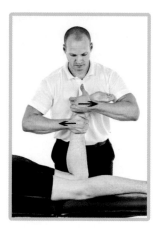

- The patient is in the prone position.
- Stand to the side of the table, on the side you will be manipulating.
- Flex the knee to 90°.
- Place your right hand around the distal tibia and fibula as close to the tibiotalar joint as possible.
- Place your left hand around the posterior aspect of the calcaneus.
- Ask the patient to inhale and exhale.
- Halfway through the exhalation phase, begin to engage the barrier by pulling your hands apart and towards your sternum.
- To manipulate the joint, perform a rapid pulling-apart motion of the hands while bringing your elbows to your side.

### Key Points
- Ensure that the table is at the correct height, so that with the knee flexed to 90° the patient's foot is level with the middle of your sternum.
- To increase the speed of the manipulation, you should concentrate on making the movement of your elbows to your side as fast as possible.

## Crouching Subtalar Manipulation

- The patient is in supine position.
- Stand at the foot of the table, facing the patient, then crouch to be level with the table.
- Use an asymmetrical squat posture.
- Both 5th metacarpals are interlinked and cover the trochlear of the talus.

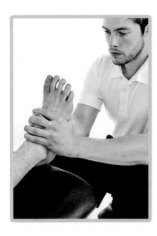
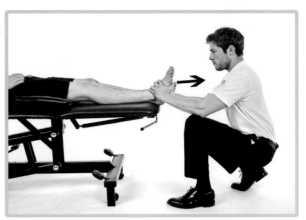

- With your lateral hand, take up the skin slack and create a lateral draw towards the 5th tarsal.
- Bring both thumbs under the plantar aspect of the foot and contact under the distal portion of the calcaneus.
- Create internal or external rotation of the limb to lock out the hip.
- Ask the patient to inhale and exhale.
- On exhalation, engage the barrier and perform the manipulation by pulling through your elbows.

**Key Points**
- Ensure good posture when crouching down.
- Keep your elbows tight into the body, posture upright and weight over the back foot.
- Ensure that you take all skin slack away from the contact area by using a medial draw of the fingers over the dorsal aspect of the foot.
- Allow the patient to hold on to the table to ensure that they feel comfortable and stable.

## Side-Lying Subtalar Manipulation

- Have the patient lie on the side of the foot you wish to manipulate with the knee bent at 90°.
- For the patient's comfort, place a towel underneath the lower leg.
- Adopt an asymmetrical stance.
- Adjust the height of the table to allow you to contact the patient's foot with your arms almost straight.

- Place your left hand, with a broad contact between the thumb and index finger, over the distal lower leg, as close to the talocrural joint as possible.
- Place your right hand over the PM aspect of the calcaneus.
- Ask the patient to inhale and exhale; at the end of exhalation, the barrier should be engaged.
- Perform an ML manipulation with your right hand down towards the floor.

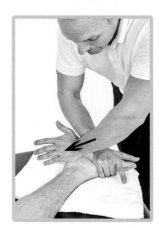

**Key Points**

- For the patient's comfort, place a towel underneath the foot.
- The stabilising hand does just that. There is no need to thrust with this hand.
- Use of a drop piece (if one is available with your table) is very effective in this situation as it can reduce the amount of force needed.

## Side-Lying Subtalar Manipulation Variation

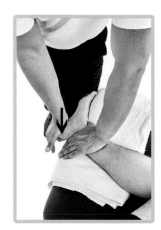

- Have the patient lie on the side of the foot you wish to manipulate with the knee bent at 90°; the foot should be hanging just over the side of the table.
- Stand at the side of the table, facing towards it.
- Adjust the height of the table to allow you to contact the patient's foot with arms almost straight.
- Place your left hand, with a broad contact between the thumb and index finger, over the distal lower leg, as close to the talocrural joint as possible.
- Place your right hand over the PM aspect of the calcaneus
- Ask the patient to inhale and exhale; at the end of exhalation, the barrier should be engaged.

- Perform an ML manipulation with your right hand down towards the floor.

**Key Points**
- For the patient's comfort, place a towel underneath the foot.
- The stabilising hand does just that. There is no need to thrust with this hand.
- Use of a drop piece (if one is available with your table) is very effective in this situation as it can reduce the amount of force needed.

# Standing Subtalar Manipulation

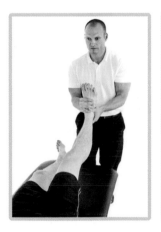 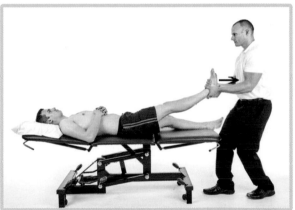

- The patient is in supine position.
- Stand at foot of table, facing the patient, with an asymmetrical stance.
- Your left hand contacts the calcaneus and your right hand contacts the trochlear of the talus with your 5th metacarpal.
- Use the thumb of your right hand to create a slight dorsiflexion of the ankle.
- Create internal or external rotation of the limb to lock out the hip and decrease the movement potential of the joint.
- Ask the patient to inhale and exhale.
- At the end of the exhalation phase, engage the barrier and manipulate the joint.
- The manipulation is achieved by pulling your elbows sharply towards you and leaning on to your back foot to use your body weight.

### Key Points

- Keep your elbows tight into your body and your posture upright, and drop your body weight down on to your back foot to create tension and traction through the joints.
- The thrust should be a combination of body power and arm speed, rather than just a 'pull' through the arms.
- Allow the patient to hold on to the table to ensure that they feel comfortable and stable.

## Prone Talocalcaneal Manipulation

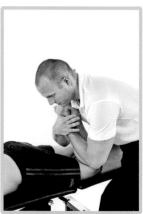

- Have the patient in a prone position with the ankle to be manipulated closest to the side of the couch. (The image shows the left ankle being manipulated so the technique is performed on your right side.)
- Flex the knee up to 90° to allow you to take hold of the calcaneus between the thumb and forefinger of both hands.
- Your hands will fit tightly against the posterior aspect of the calcaneus.
- Rest the anterior aspect of the foot over your shoulder.
- As you stand up, move posterior and obliquely to bring on a slight traction to the talocalcaneal joint.
- The patient is asked to inhale and exhale.
- Halfway through the exhalation phase, engage the barrier.
- The manipulation is given through your legs; your arms are there to stabilise the joint. When you reach the barrier of the joint, stand up, performing the manipulation in an SO direction.

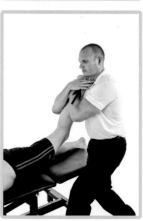

**Key Points**

- This technique should be avoided if the patient has any instability in the knee or hip, or if they have acute lumbar pain, as this is a long-lever technique and can transfer force through adjoining structures.
- A towel can be placed on your shoulder for the patient's comfort.
- The manipulation should be performed as the patient exhales.
- Ensure you reach the barrier before applying the manipulation in order to minimise the force being distributed through other structures.

# Talocalcaneal Manipulation

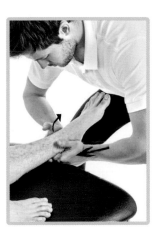

- Ask the patient to lie in the supine position.
- Stand at the foot of the table, facing towards the patient, with an asymmetrical stance.
- With your fingers pointing towards the floor, your left hand contacts the calcaneus on both sides as shown.
- Your left hand is over the medial aspect of the calcaneonavicular joint.
- Your right hand is in contact with the distal fibula so that your fingers rest above the fingers of the hand gripping the calcaneus.
- Ask the patient to inhale and exhale, and engage the barrier.
- Once the barrier is engaged, perform the manipulation is a movement from ML with your right hand.
- At the same time your left hand contacting the distal fibula is manipulated PA.

**Key Points**

- Ask the patient to let the foot go slack.
- The technique is used to increase calcaneal eversion.
- Thrust with both hands simultaneously to ensure maximal distraction between the calcaneus and the navicular.

## Talonavicular Manipulation

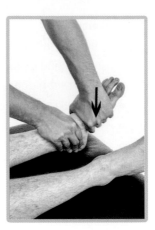

- Ask the patient to lie in the supine position.
- Adopt an asymmetrical stance on the ipsilateral side of the table, facing the foot you are manipulating.
- Both arms need to be near full extension at the elbow.
- With your left hand, place your index finger on the navicular tuberosity.
- Stabilise the patient's distal tibia/fibula with a broad-based contact, using your right hand as shown.
- Ask the patient to inhale and exhale.
- At the end of exhalation, engage the barrier by pronating the foot via the navicular with slight plantar flexion.
- Once you have engaged the barrier, perform the manipulation with a short, sharp, fast movement incorporating the pronation and slight plantar flexion.

### Key Points

- Speed is key: the quicker the thrust, the less force needed.
- Use your non-contact hand only to stabilise.

## Mid-Foot Manipulation (Talonavicular and Navicular Cuneiforms)

- The patient is in the supine position.
- Approach the bench and hold the working foot in both hands.
- Stand at the foot of table facing patient, using an asymmetrical stance.
- With the 5th metacarpal of your right hand, cover the trochlear of the talus.
- Your left hand holds on to the calcaneus.

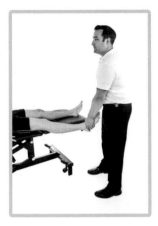
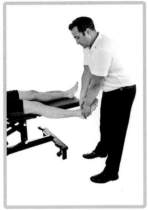
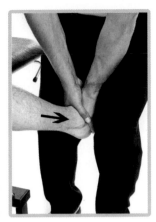

- Create internal or external rotation of the limb to lock out the hip.
- Ask the patient to inhale and exhale.
- On the exhalation phase, engage the barrier and perform the manipulation by pulling through your elbows.

**Key Points**
- Reverse the above for the other foot.
- To manipulate the cuneiforms, move your hand from the trochlear of the talus to the row of cuneiforms.
- Keep your elbows tight into the body, posture upright and weight over the back foot.
- Allow the patient to hold on to the table to ensure that they feel comfortable and stable.

# Navicular Manipulation

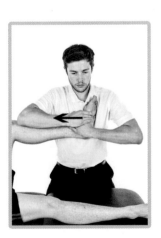

- The patient is in the supine position.
- Stand on the ipsilateral side of the table to the side you are manipulating.
- With the knee and hip flexed to 90°, the foot is roughly level with the middle of your sternum.
- Your left hand contacts over the talocrural joint with all five fingers, resting the palm of your hand over the medial aspect of the patient's calcaneus.

- Your right hand is over the medial aspect of the foot so that the 1st, 4th and 5th fingers are relaxed and resting over the plantar aspect.
- The contact point for the manipulation is the PIP of the 3rd finger. Ensure that when positioning the contact hand this joint is in contact with the navicular tuberosity.
- To complete set-up, ensure that the forearm of the contact hand is parallel and resting lightly on the shin of the patient's leg.
- Ask the patient to inhale and exhale. At the end of exhalation, engage the barrier.
- To manipulate the joint. perform a rapid pulling-apart motion of the hands while bringing your elbows to your side.

### Key Points
- To increase the speed of the adjustment, you should concentrate on making the movement of your elbows to your side as fast as possible.

## Prone Cuboid Manipulation

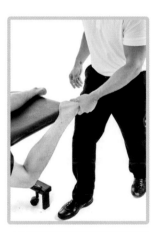

- The patient lies prone, slightly off centre and closer to the side of the table you are standing on.
- Hold the foot with both hands and adopt an asymmetrical stance.
- Bring the affected foot off the table, allowing knee and hip flexion.
- Contact over the lateral border of the foot and palpate the cuboid.
- Your left thumb covers the posterior aspect of the cuboid; support your thumb with the other thumb crossed over.
- Ask the patient to inhale and exhale.
- Towards the end of the exhalation phase, engage the barrier.

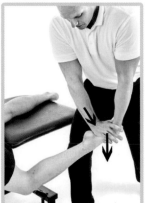

- Keeping your body weight directly over the points of contact, manipulate downward and slightly oblique.
- The manipulation occurs from a slight extension of both arms and a small forward movement through your legs.

**Key Points**
- This technique can be used over both the medial and the lateral borders.
- While trying to engage the barrier, you can use momentum by adding slight hip and knee flexion.

## Phalangeal Manipulation

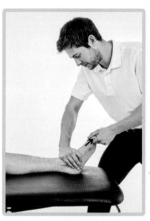

- The patient is in the supine position.
- Adopt an asymmetrical stance.
- Your right hand stabilises over the talonavicular joint.
- Your left hand contacts the toe between the thumb and palm.
- Ask the patient to inhale and exhale. At the end of exhalation, engage the barrier.
- Perform the manipulation by pulling towards you.

**Key Points**
- This technique is applicable to all toes.
- Keep your body weight just behind the ankle, contact hand elbow tucked into the side.

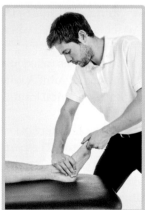

# Glossary

**Abduction** Movement of an outlying joint away from the midline.

**Active motion** Patient's voluntary movement.

**AC joint** Acromioclavicular joint.

**Adduction** Movement of an outlying joint towards the midline.

**Amplitude** Distance of articulation.

**Anterior** Near or towards the front.

**Anterior-posterior (AP)** Direction from front to back.

**Appendicular skeleton** The part of the skeleton consisting of the bones or cartilage that support the appendages.

**Applicator** A part of the operator's body which is placed on the contact point of the patient.

**Anterior-superior (AS)** Direction from front to up.

**Arthrokinematics** The specific simultaneous movement of joint surfaces (classed as roll, glide and spin). Sometimes also called arthrokinematic movement or joint play.

**Articular process** Small flat projections on either side of a vertebra incorporating the articular surface.

**Asymmetrical stance** One foot in front of the other.

**Articulation** Place where two or more bones unite. Also, the active or passive progress of moving a joint through its allowed physiological range of motion. Sometimes called joint mobilisation.

**Atlantoaxial joint** A joint between the first and second cervical vertebrae.

**Atlanto-occipital joint** A synovial joint between the occiput and the first cervical vertebra.

**Atlas** The first cervical vertebra.

**Axial skeleton** The part of the skeleton that consists of the bones of the head and trunk.

**Axis** The second cervical vertebra.

**Biaxial** Having two axes.

**Biaxial joint** A joint in which the rounded surface of an oval bone fits within a cup-shaped socket on the other bone, allowing movements in two planes.

**Bilateral** Involving two or both sides.

**Brevis** Brief or short.

**Bursa** A fluid-filled sac that serves to reduce friction between a bone and the surrounding soft tissue.

**Caudal/caudad** Towards the tail/inferiorly.

**Cavitation** Refers to the formation and activity of gaseous bubbles (or cavities) within the synovial fluid of a joint.

**Cervical (C)** Neck.

**Circumduction** The active or passive movement of a limb in a circular fashion (e.g. the circular motion of the ball-and-socket joint).

**Coccyx** Tip or end of the tailbone.

**Collagen** The main structural protein in the connective tissues.

**Condyle** The rounded articular prominence at the end of a bone.

**Contact point** The part of the patient's body where the operator places the applicator.

**Contraction** A process in which muscle tension is increased, with or without change in overall length.

**Contralateral** On the opposite side.

**Coronal/frontal** Plane dividing the body into anterior and posterior parts by passing through it longitudinally from one side to the other.

**Coronal axis** A horizontal line extending from left to right. Flexion and extension movements usually occur around this axis.

**Cranial/cephalad/cephalic** Towards the head/superiorly.

**Crack** An audible sound that signifies a successful application of a manipulative procedure.

**Crepitation** An audible crackling or rattling sound or feeling during movement of tendons or ligaments over bone.

**Cross fibre/kneading** Soft-tissue technique: intermittent force that is applied transversely to the long axis of muscle.

**Deep pressure/inhibition** Soft-tissue technique: a local sustained force that is applied to a specific joint.

**Deltoid muscle** Thick, triangular-shaped muscle covering the shoulder.

**Deviation** Movement of the joint either laterally or medially from the anatomical midline.

**DIP joint** Distal interphalangeal joint.

**Distal** Further from the centre or the point of origin.

**Distraction** Force acting along a perpendicular to longitudinal axis to draw the structures apart.

**Dorsal** Relating to the back of the hand or the top surface of the foot.

**Effleurage** Soft-tissue technique: a stroking movement performed in order to encourage the return of fluid from distal to proximal.

**Epicondyle** A rounded eminence above the condyle of a long bone.

**Eversion** Foot-related movement in a lateral direction.

**Extension** Backward motion in a sagittal plane about a transverse axis. Straightening of a spinal curve (exception: cervical and lumbar spines) or internal angle.

**Fascia** The soft-tissue component of the connective tissue system extending over the whole body just below the skin.

**Fibrous joint** A joint connected by fibrous connective tissue.

**Flexion** Bending movement that decreases a spinal curve (exception: thoracic spine) and internal angle.

**Frontal plane** A vertical plane through the longitudinal axis, dividing the body into anterior and posterior parts.

**Gapping** Medial and lateral – opening one side of a joint.

**Genu valgum** A physical deformity in which the distal end of the distal bone is laterally displaced in the joint.

**Genu varum** A physical deformity in which the distal end of the distal bone is medially displaced in the joint.

**Hypaxial** Below the centre line, axis.

**Hypoalgesia** Decreased sensitivity to pain.

**Hypothenar eminence** A muscular protrusion at the medial side of the palm which controls the movement of the little finger.

**Hypertonicity** A condition of unusually high muscle tension.

**HVLA** High-velocity, low-amplitude (see *Manipulation*).

**Impulse** A sudden forceful push or driving force.

**Inferior (inf)** Bottom.

**Inferior-medial (IM)** Direction from bottom to nearer the midline of the body.

**Inferior-superior (IS)** Direction from bottom to top.

**Insertion** The site of attachment of a muscle to the part to be moved.

**Interstitial** The space between structures.

**Inversion** Foot-related movement in a medial direction.

**Ipsilateral** On the same side.

**Kinetic** Relating to motion.

**Kyphosis** An abnormal increase in posterior convexity of the spine.

**Lateral (lat)** Further away from the midline.

**Lateral flexion** Movement in a coronal (frontal) plane about an anterior–posterior axis. Also called side-bending.

**Longitudinal stretch** Soft-tissue technique: stretch force that is applied along the long axis of muscle.

**Lordosis** Abnormally increased anteroposterior curvature of the spine.

**Lower extremity** Thigh, leg and foot.

**Lumbar (L)** Lower back.

**Manipulation** A type of manual therapy in which a thrust is applied to the patient in order to produce mechanical responses (see *HVLA*).

**Mechanoreceptor** A sensory receptor that responds to mechanical stimuli.

**MCP joint** Metacarpophalangeal joint.

**Medial** (**med**) Closer to the midline.

**Medial-lateral** (**ML**) From toward the middle to the outside.

**Meniscoid** Intercapsular synovial fold formed either in the embryo or as a result of trauma to the joint.

**Mobilisation** See *Articulation*.

**Musculature** The muscular system of a body or region of the body.

**Multiaxial** A ball-and-socket joint that allows an extensive mobility in almost all directions.

**Nerve** A group of long, thin fibres that transmits sensory or motor information to the brain.

**Neuralgia** Severe or intense pain along the pathway of a nerve.

**Neurotransmitters** Potential brain chemicals involved in the modulation of pain perception.

**Nociceptor** Sensory receptor (neuron) that sends signals to cause the perception of pain in response to potentially damaging stimuli.

**Nociception** The sensation of pain due to neural processing of a harmful stimulus.

**Oblique-posterior** (**OP**) From a sloping direction to nearer the rear.

**Occiput** (**O**) The back of the head or skull.

**Operator** Practitioner, therapist.

**Orthopaedics** A branch of medicine that deals with the diagnosis and treatment of musculoskeletal diseases.

**Osteoporosis** Atrophy of bone tissue, resulting from hormonal changes or lack of calcium or vitamin D.

**Ossification** The process of transforming cartilage into a bony material.

**Osteokinematics** The basic movements of a joint (e.g. flexion, extension, abduction, adduction). Sometimes also called osteokinematic movement or physiologic movement.

**Palmar** Palm surface of the hand.

**Passive motion** Movement made by the operator while the patient is relaxed or passive.

**Patient** Individual receiving treatment.

**Paraphysiological space** The space or zone of elasticity between the physiologic barrier and the anatomic barrier.

**Parietal** Relating to the walls of a cavity.

**Paraesthesia** Pins-and-needles sensation.

**Paraspinal muscles** Muscles that are adjacent to the vertebral column.

**Plantar** Sole surface of the foot.

**Plicae** Embryological synovial folds that occur mainly in the knee joint.

**Posterior** (**post**) Back.

**Posterior-anterior** (**PA**) Direction from back to front.

**Posterior-anterior-superior** (**PAS**) From back to front with an upward movement.

**Posterior-inferior** (**PI**) Direction from back to bottom.

**Posterior-medial** (**PM**) Direction from back to middle.

**PIP joint** Proximal interphalangeal joint.

**Pronation** Applied to the hand: an act of turning the palmer surface/medial rotation. Applied to the foot: a combination of abduction or eversion in the tarsal or metatarsal joints.

**Proximal** Situated nearer to the origin of a point of attachment.

**Quadrangular** Having four angles.

**Quadriceps** The large group of muscle at the front of the thigh that includes four distinct parts.

**Receptor** A structure on the cell surface that receives stimuli.

**Reinforce** Applying extra pressure in order to focus specifically on or protect another part of the body by placing the applicator.

**Retraction** The act of withdrawing or drawing back.

**Reflexogenic** Causing a reflex effect.

**ROM** Range of motion.

**Rotation** Movement about an axis – internal, external or medial, lateral.

**Sacroiliac joints** Joints between the sacrum and the ilia.

**Sacrum** Tail bone between the two halves of the pelvis.

**Sagittal** Plane dividing the body into left and right portions by passing through it longitudinally from the front to the back.

**Scoliosis** Abnormally increased lateral deviation of the spine.

**Shearing** Action or force inclining to lead to two adjoining parts of an articulation to slide in the direction of their plane of contact relative to each other.

**Shifting** Anteroposterior (A/P) and lateral (Lat). Sliding movement.

**Side-bending** See *Lateral flexion*.

**Soft tissue** Tissue other than bone or joint.

**Springing** Application of repetitive and subtle force to a targeted point.

**Superior** (**sup**) Top.

**Superior-inferior** (**SI**) Direction from top to bottom.

**Superior-oblique** (**SO**) From top to a slanting position.

**Superficial** Nearer to the body surface.

**Supination** Applied to the hand: turning the palm forward or upward by lateral external rotation of the forearm. Applied to the foot: applying adduction and inversion movement to the medial margin of the foot.

**Superior-posterior** (**SP**) Direction from top to back.

**Sprain** Tearing or stretching of ligaments and/or tendons of a joint.

**SC joint** Sternoclavicular joint.

**Symmetrical stance** Feet are side by side.

**Syndesmosis** An immovable joint bound by interosseous ligaments.

**Symphyses** A fusion between two articulating bones separated by pad of fibrocartilage.

**Synergism** The working together of two or more organs, tissues or joints to generate a combined effect.

**Synovial** A type of joint that contains a lubricating substance (synovial fluid) and is lined with a thick flexible membrane.

**Synovial fold** A pleat of the synovial membrane located on the inner surface of the joint capsule.

**Tactile** Pertaining to the sense of touch.

**Thenar eminence** The lateral side of the hand palmar surface heel.

**Thoracic (T)/dorsal (D)** Mid and upper back.

**Thorax** The region of the body located between the neck and the abdomen.

**Thrust** An external force applied during manipulation.

**Traction** Force acting along a longitudinal axis in order to draw the structures apart.

**Translation** Motion along an axis.

**Transverse** Plane dividing the body to upper and lower portions by passing perpendicular to sagittal and frontal planes horizontally through the body.

**Trunk** The part of the human body extending from the neck to pelvic region.

**TVP or TP** Transverse process.

**Upper extremity** Arm, forearm and hand.

**Unilateral** Pertaining to one side of a structure.

**Vascular** Relating to vessels or ducts that convey blood and lymph.

**Visceral** Relating to the viscera or the internal organs of the body.

**Ventral** See *Anterior*.

**Zygapophysial joints** A set of synovial joints formed by joining the superior and inferior articular processes.

# Subject Index

# Author Index